My Brain Can't Poop:
A mental fitness guide for humans

SCOTT MIKESH

DEDICATION

Unless you have a bar code printed on your behind, you likely weren't born with an operator's manual. So I dedicate this book to YOU—dear human—for making your brain health and mental fitness a priority, to make the most of this life that you have (with no extended warranty)!

What makes life especially challenging is how we're all trying to figure ourselves out as we go—inside and out—all at the same time, day after day, year after year, moment to moment, for as many moments as we have. One of the most challenging bits about life is that there never seem to be enough of those moments. When time seems to fly, it can sure add to our stress and impatience, that can significantly impact our brain health and function (that we'll talk about a whole lot more).

Time seems especially fleeting when we fail to pay conscious attention to each moment, because we neither live in the future nor in the past. All we ever really have is this present moment that is right now—that is life. Due to the very slight delay in your conscious response, however, the very instant you are consciously aware of this moment, the moment has passed, and a new moment already took its place—over, and over, and over again. Every moment seems to pass as quickly as we realize it.

A major reason why being mentally present in the moment you are living can be so difficult is due to how your brain responds to stress, that is faster than your conscious comprehension.

Since we never know what tomorrow will bring, and we cannot change the past, we can trigger stress in ourselves when all we think about is what was or what might be. This stress response further delays our conscious awareness from focusing on the present moment.

Arguably so, this present moment is the most precious non-renewable resource of all, that is yours to do with as you see fit—to experience, explore, and enjoy—to make the most of the life you have with the abilities you have, as well as you can for as long as you can. The very best you can do is use each invaluable moment to learn, heal, develop, plan, and prepare—including those essential moments of rest and recovery you need to feel and do your best..

Thank you for sharing this incredibly valuable moment with me, that I do not take for granted.

Your brain, body, and life experiences are all as unique as you are, and the only person who really knows and understands them all as intimately as you do is you. It takes time and patience to explore, discover, and accept yourself—inside and out—to find the care and support you need to feel and do your best. Only you can figure yourself out and navigate your life as it unfolds around you.

However you identify as a human being, this book was written for you. Your very human brain needs and deserves as much attention, understanding, and care as every other, to get what you want out of every moment you have.

I also want to dedicate this book to all those who have and continue to encourage and embrace self-discovery, wonderment, exploration, encouragement, and acceptance, by asking questions and seeking answers, challenging and being challenged, that's all essential to human growth and development.

Most of all, I am grateful for all of you healthful humans who invest your time and energy to reduce unhealthful stress, fear, and shame in yourself and others; that is the key to unlocking your full human potential.

As with any fitness workout or training program, I hope this book challenges you in healthful ways as you learn more about your brain and the brains of others, to keep growing and developing mentally and physically, to feel and do your best to achieve your goals.

I hope your mind does a few flips along the way as you think about fitness differently, by prioritizing your brain health and mental well-being with preventive care and proactive practices, as you keep learning, exploring, growing, and discovering— moment to moment, inside and out—practicing and preparing for the many mental and emotional challenges of life.

By the end, I hope you feel more empowered and aware of the healthful influences you need to optimize and maintain your motivation to succeed. Even when the most challenging step you can take is just waking up to face the day, remember that every step counts toward achieving your goals, no matter how big or small.

Whether this is your first step or your one-millionth, I want you to believe in yourself and your abilities, what you can do when you have healthful information, guidance, representation, understanding, rest, nourishment, exercise, resources, and support—to care for your brain as best you can. This is really what fitness is all about.

Thank you for joining this mental fitness movement as we keep learning about ourselves and each other along the way!

CONTENTS

"When we dismiss or deny the function of the brain, we prolong the cycle of dysfunction and pain."

PREFACE

Prioritize your mental health

We interrupt your regularly scheduled reading for this important healthcare reminder, to prioritize your mental health.

Your mind is a critical function of your brain that is connected to every neurological and physiological system in your body, and influenced by everything inside and outside of your body as well. It's important to remember that just as any physical fitness program is not a substitute or replacement for physical healthcare, neither is any mental fitness program a replacement for mental healthcare, that might include routine check-ups, therapy, or counseling services to maintain your overall health and well-being.

Fitness practices provide proactive and preventive ways to supplement and support your overall health, so it's still important to consult your mental or physical healthcare provider(s) before making any changes to your lifestyle, health habits, physical activity, nutrition, or body chemistry to avoid any unintended consequences of making changes that could impact your overall health outcomes and coordination of care. It's always in your best interest to have all those who are caring for you on the same page as they aim for the same goal of helping you feel and do your best physically, mentally, and emotionally.

The ultimate aim of mental fitness is to empower you to make your own brain health and mental well-being a priority. This not only includes practices that can help you feel and do your best, but also greater awareness of the mental, emotional, and physical signals your brain and body send that indicate imbalance, illness, injury, trauma, loss, or impairment, that may require more specialized care and attention.

You DESERVE to feel and do your best with the care and healing you need. If you need more specialized care, please speak with your primary doctor or contact a mental healthcare provider in your area to find the care, treatment, or therapeutic services you need to balance or heal your neurology and physiology.

If you are experiencing thoughts, feelings, or behaviors that are getting in the way of you feeling and doing your best in your daily activities, relationships, education, career, goals, etc. you may have a mental health condition (or even more than one) that is at the root of it. Just as you would seek proper care for a physical imbalance, illness, injury, trauma, loss, or impairment, so must mental health conditions be properly identified and treated by a licensed mental healthcare professional who can help you heal or manage your health in a healthful way.

Since mental healthcare largely depends on you sharing your inner-most thoughts and deepest personal feelings, a sense of trust and safety between you and your healthcare provider is essential to providing proper care.

Diagnosing an injury, illness, imbalance, or impairment doesn't involve finding the spot that feels good, but finding the spot that hurts, in order to understand why, to provide proper care. While it may be emotionally painful to acknowledge the source of your pain (that is very much neurological, much like touching a bruise), adding to the pain or ignoring it is not what stops or heals it, any more than physical pain.

Similar to physical pain, you must identify and gently remove or heal what's causing your pain. This often requires specialized care and healing with the support of a healthcare practitioner.

Please know that there is nothing inherently "wrong" with how you feel, based on your neurology and physiology, and that you have every right and responsibility to be understood and cared for in a healthful and healing way.

What does cause harm is when we let our fear get in the way by neglecting or ignoring (i.e., fighting or fleeing) the challenging realities of brain health and function. We suffer even more when we don't seek and receive the care and healing we need.

There's also a reason why "courage" is part of the word "encouragement"; when you prioritize your own mental health, you become a healthful example for others who might be struggling too. Your courage to face and shed any fears you have in seeking or receiving care provides encouragement for others to courageously shed whatever fear or shame that is in their way to seek and receive care as well.

When you seek mental health services, please feel empowered and encouraged to share and explain your personal thoughts, feelings, and experiences to advocate for your own health and well-being. This is probably the most important and courageous step you will ever take to get the most out of the life that you have, by shedding the fear and shame that too often get in the way.

If ever you are experiencing a life-threatening situation, including harmful thoughts or feelings toward yourself or others, please seek immediate medical assistance by going to your nearest **Emergency Room** or **call 9-1-1** (in the U.S.), call **1-800-273-TALK (8255)** or **text "MHA" to 741741** to speak with a trained Crisis Counselor.

INTRODUCTION

As a human being, you are amazing! You may not even consciously realize how amazing you are since approximately 90 percent of your brain activity is unconscious, including most of your thoughts, feelings, and behaviors, that require little to no conscious awareness or effort on your part.

It's true! And there's an important reason why your brain and body operate unconsciously for your own health, safety, and well-being.

Imagine if you had to consciously focus on every breath and heartbeat, every little sound you heard near and far, every surface you touched including the ground and your clothing, every step or movement you made throughout your day, as well as everything you saw, smelled, or otherwise sensed in your environment.

Researchers estimate the human brain processes around eleven million bits of information unconsciously every second of every day—whether you're asleep or awake—while the conscious mind can only handle 40 to 50 bits of information per second.

Without your unconscious mind, you wouldn't be able to focus on anything else without getting distracted or forgetting to breathe or make your heart beat… beat… beat… beat… beat… don't forget to breathe!

Not to mention the amount of energy it would take your brain to operate in that way all day every day.

Talk about multitasking (I'm exhausted just thinking about it!).

Thankfully, the human brain and body send neurochemical

signals to and from one to the other unconsciously through a special part of your nervous system that requires no conscious effort on your part, and therefore uses less energy too.

This is why when you are scared or even surprised you jump, scream, or shake automatically before you consciously know what's going on... WHO?! WHAT?! WHERE?!

Immediately your heart starts to race, you breathe faster, your body starts to sweat, and you get a sudden burst of energy (powered by *adrenaline*) in preparation to fight or flee. All of this happens without any conscious effort on your part, and you can thank your brain for that!

This is where I'll mention how I really don't like surprise parties either, because of the stress response involved, which is why I think there should always be a first responder on stand-by (or at least a clean pair of underpants).

It doesn't matter if what startled you was a "real" threat or not, only that your unconscious nervous system perceived it by sending neurological signals to your brain faster than your conscious brain could comprehend it. Whether it was a hungry lion or your sadistic family and friends hiding in the dark, it doesn't matter to your nervous system—your brain still perceives those neurological signals as a threat just the same, triggering an unconscious stress response.

Your unconscious stress response really is your natural defense system that is intended to protect you from harm (which is why I advise positioning anyone who doesn't want to get punched in the face farthest away from the guest of horror... sorry, I mean guest of honor, if you think it's honorable to pee your pants).

On the other hand, your unconscious stress response can also inhibit the part of your brain responsible for comprehension, critical thinking, and problem solving, which is why talking about the brain can also seem very intimidating, complex, and confusing when we're not taught in ways that reduce our stress response, without worry of being tested and getting everything right (that ironically inhibits the part of the brain that powers comprehension). Since science is really about trial and error that requires time and patience to learn as we go, that is what we'll focus on in this book.

What I don't want you to do is stress or worry about all of the scientific jargon (especially if you hated biology and chemistry in school that might trigger an unconscious stress response and make your eyes glaze over). Besides, all of those Latin-based words that other people made up a long time ago are not the most important part of understanding how your brain works anyway.

Whether or not you remember the fancy names of all the different neurochemicals flowing through your body does not make them more or less real. The most important part is for you to develop a better sense and understanding of how your brain and body work together in everyday life, in whatever terms make the most sense to you (which is why I often use metaphors and real-life examples), including how your brain health and mental function are influenced by everything you think, feel, hear, see, view, read, touch, taste, smell, and eat. The ultimate aim is for you to feel empowered to ask questions and seek what you need to feel and do your best—without fear, stress, shame, or worry—by prioritizing your brain health and mental well-being, because you are a human who needs and deserves it.

While dreams and positive thoughts can help to a point (by reducing stress and fueling motivation), as we become increasingly stressed and distracted, and decreasingly hopeful and patient in our faster-is-better instant-gratification information-overload lifestyle—especially when we're fueled by the fear of losing, missing out, or running out of time—dreaming and positive thinking alone are not enough.

We must first understand brain function to optimize it, with mental fitness practices that promote brain health and mental well-being neurologically and physiologically.

Why, you ask? That's a great question we need to keep asking!

The most important lesson to learn, even before you take that first step toward your goal, is to develop the perception that you are important, valuable, and significant. We often take for granted that we should all immediately feel this way about ourselves, but for most of us, it is not that easy, because of how our brains work—neurologically and physiologically—and everything that influences our thoughts and feelings, inside and out.

Unless you have someone else who can help calm your fear and reassure you that you matter, that your health and well-being matters, it's very hard to convince ourselves of this fact, when our unconscious mind and emotions tell us otherwise.

There is nothing quite as frightening, intimidating, or overwhelming than a sense of emptiness, an endless void of nothingness, with a general lack of direction, purposes, and support. That may be why finding purpose in life is such a focal point for mental well-being, but stating the obvious isn't always helpful unless you learn how to do it.

You may have every intention and desire to make healthful choices, to make a healthful difference, to find meaning and purpose, to feel confident and motivated, yet still feel a sense of emptiness, hopelessness, or meaninglessness that defeats you before you even get started.

These are the ugly and frightening feelings associated with

anxiety and depression, very real and serious neurological and physiological health conditions.

Feelings (both sensations and emotions) are a result of neurochemical activity that act as signals to inform us where we are and where we need to go, like an internal guidance system. Just like every other part of our biological system, sometimes our neurological system needs to be healed or rebalanced with proper care and adjustment.

As a human, you are not a simple mechanical machine, but a highly complex organism that is an important part of our natural world. You deserve proper care and protection, just like every other part of nature.

So, let's talk about your human brain and mental function in an easy-to-understand (low stress) way. Consider this book a general guide and starting point for your mental fitness practice. The first half is all about brain function and mental influences, and the second half is all about the progressive levels of mental fitness and practices you can use to optimize brain health and mental function, to help you feel and do your best. Feel free to jump around and choose the sections that most interest you, or read in sequence all the way through for the most comprehensive overview.

We'll cover basic brain function to help you learn how and why different mental fitness practices work, to decide what works best for you and your brain. There is no need to remember every complex term or physiological process, as long as you grasp the basic concepts you need to understand how to care for your brain, to feel and do your best. (I highly encourage you to do more research about any topic that you find of interest, for your own brain health and mental fitness practice!)

Every step counts on the path toward achieving your goals, so consider this one of them!

For me personally, I knew that writing this book would be a serious mental fitness practice in itself, and that it sure was. Not only was it a challenge to sift and articulate information and ideas in a coherent way, but the stress was compounded by the immense community health and safety crises that erupted during the COVID-19 pandemic.

As I'm sure yours are too, my thoughts and feelings have been utterly consumed by the pandemic, political protests and civil unrest, along with the sudden halt to my business, that resulted in an extended period of unemployment (not to mention a serious craving for banana bread, and a nearly non-existent desire to exercise).

While partly written during one of the most challenging times of our lifetime, my hope is that this book will be a source of hope and motivation for you as much as it has been for me—like a light at the end of the tunnel, to make the most of the life you have.

After years of studying psychology, design, and mass media, and decades of applying my knowledge and skills in marketing and communications, health and wellness, and D.E.I. (diversity, equity, and inclusion), I realized how much effort is made and paid to influence attitudes and behaviors when it comes to producing, performing, selling, buying, voting, consuming, watching, clicking, eating, drinking, looking good, etc.—often with little understanding or consideration of brain health, or how thoughts, attitudes, and behaviors are influenced in less-than-healthful ways, every moment of every day.

I also found that many well-meaning efforts to influence healthful behaviors lack general awareness and understanding of the competing influences that make healthful behaviors so hard to achieve and maintain, often overlooking and neglecting brain health and function in exchange for fast (and temporary) results.

I found there to be very little awareness or consideration of diverse brain function and mental conditions that affect different people in different ways as well, with little to no awareness of how difficult and complicated even healthful changes can be mentally, emotionally, and physically for many people—especially with so much shame and stigma directed at those who struggle.

We give labels to people and conditions in order to maintain a sense of control, order, and understanding (since we tend to fear the unknown), but people are neither static nor one-dimensional as most labels imply. We are complex beings with complex thoughts, feelings, identities, ideas, and life experiences. We are constantly changing, growing, developing, and adapting in ways we most often are not even aware.

Rather than relying on labels alone (that change over time too), my aim is to cultivate a greater sense of safety and understanding through thoughtful conversation and self-discovery, with personal disclosure neither forced nor discouraged. Every person must feel empowered to decide for themselves when, how, what, and with whom they want to share their inner-most thoughts and feelings—in their own time, in their own way—to allow every person to feel and do their best.

I developed my mental fitness programs to focus on the mind as a vital function of the brain, which impacts every aspect of life, including your ability to care and create, to learn and communicate, to relate and feel comfortable in your own skin.

In this modern age, we are bombarded by information and stimulation in profound ways. All that we absorb through our senses impacts how we perceive the world—how we think, feel, and behave.

More than ever, media, apps, and entertainment are influencing our thoughts, feelings, and actions, to consume, click, buy, vote, subscribe, crave, and compete; sometimes passively, sometimes interactively, and sometimes addictively.

Not that all tech and media are bad, because it's an important part of our culture and economy. Technology is also used to educate and entertain in ways that promote healthful thoughts, feelings, and behaviors, offering helpful information, guidance, and support.

The information we consume is like any other part of our environment that we must be aware of and care about, to promote healthful outcomes and avoid unhealthful effects, the same as we care about the air we breathe, the water we drink, and the food we eat.

Maintaining the health of our minds as a neurological and physiological function of our brains requires the same care and commitment as maintaining the health of our bodies, because while our body is the vehicle, our mind is the driver—both consciously and unconsciously.

In this fast-paced world, though, it's getting harder to take care of our brains and bodies. We're working longer hours with less time off. We've been sold on the idea that faster is better. We barely allow enough time to sleep and eat, and we feel guilty for slowing down, worrying about everything that needs to get done. We struggle to find the time and energy for healthy physical activity, and we eat food that is fast and easy, that lacks nutrition; and it's deteriorating our health.

What makes things trickier is that we have developed and manufactured so many chemicals and artificial ingredients that we now know do us more harm than good, and lack the essential nutrients we need. Of course, we learned all of this after they become staples in our lives, after our habits had formed and our cravings had been conditioned.

So now, not only do we need to practice healthful habits, but we also need to sift through information about everything we consume physically and mentally—that is most often hard-to-find and verify—in order to determine the short term and long-term effects on our natural human physiology and neurology, in order to find those that are the most healthful, sustainable, and beneficial for our human brains and bodies.

According to the National Research Council and Institute of Medicine, Americans have a shorter life expectancy compared to almost all other high-income countries, and up to half of all premature (or early) deaths in the United States are due to behavioral and other preventable factors.

From an article published in 2008 by the National Center for Biotechnology Information (NCBI) titled *Life Events, Stress and Illness*:

"The relationship between stress and illness is complex. Our immune system is susceptible to stress, and the susceptibility to stress varies from person to person. An event that causes an illness in a person may not cause illness in another person. Events must interact with a wide variety of background factors to manifest as an illness. Among the factors that influenced the susceptibility to stress are genetic vulnerability, coping style, type of personality and social support. When we are confronted with a problem, we assess the seriousness of the problem and determine whether or not we have the resources necessary to cope with the problem. If we believe that the problem is serious and do not have the resources necessary to cope with the problem, we will perceive ourselves as being under stress. It is our way of reacting to the situations that makes a difference in our susceptibility to illness and our overall well-being.

Not all stress has negative effect. When the body tolerates stress and uses it to overcome lethargy or enhance performance, the stress is positive, healthy and challenging. Stress is positive when it forces us to adapt and thus to increase the strength of our adaptation mechanisms, warns us that we are not coping well and that a lifestyle change is warranted if we are to maintain optimal health. This action-enhancing stress gives the athlete the competitive edge and the public speaker the enthusiasm to project optimally. Stress is negative when it exceeds our ability to cope, fatigues body systems and causes behavioral or physical problems.

The morbidity and mortality due to stress-related illness is alarming. Emotional stress is a major contributing factor to the six leading causes of death in the United States: cancer, coronary heart disease, accidental injuries, respiratory disorders, cirrhosis of the liver and suicide. The Centre for Disease Control and Prevention of the United States estimates that stress accounts for about 75% of all doctor visits. This involves an extremely wide span of physical complaints including, but not limited to, headache, back pain, heart problems, upset stomach, stomach ulcer, sleep problems, tiredness, and accidents. According to Occupational Health and Safety news and the National Council on compensation of insurance, up to 90% of all visits to primary care physicians are for stress-related complaints."

And it's not only a matter of saving millions of lives, but also millions of dollars, including precious time and resources (including yours!). According to a 2016 World Health Organization report, for every $1 spent on mental healthcare, there is a return of $4 gained in health and productivity.

So the multi-million-dollar question is, knowing all of this, why are we still struggling? Why haven't we connected the dots yet? Why is doing the healthful thing so hard?

The long and the short of it is how the human brain works— that involves complex neurochemical activity—that is part of our natural stress response, which can inhibit creativity, compassion, and critical thinking as well.

When our minds and bodies are not rested, nourished, and cared for in healthy ways, we do unhealthy things to ourselves and others. We've created a toxic culture, and it's making us sick. Our life expectancy is now declining, with increasing rates of heart disease, obesity, anxiety, depression, drug abuse, and suicide.

Not only are we struggling to stay well, but we often lack the motivation to even try, because we are all too often driven by fear, the fear of failure, or the fear of success, the fear of losing our job, of not meeting expectations, of being rejected, of being alone, of not having enough, or ultimately running out of time.

We're told to be our authentic selves, often without acknowledging the pain and struggles that come along with it; and when we struggle on our own, without encouragement or support, we lose hope.

We might attempt to self-medicate to take the fear and pain away, often in unhealthy ways. We might consciously know what's harmful and unhealthy, but when we feel hopeless, ashamed, or uncertain, and don't understand the workings of our brain and body, we resort to anything that gives us a momentary relief or sense of comfort.

Now more than ever, we need greater access, education, and preventive services that apply to all people, for every state of mental health and function, as we work to shed the historical trauma, shame, and stigma that has held us back.

Focusing on mental fitness is a way to better understand how and why you think, feel, and behave the way you do, to find the healthful practices, resources, and support you need to feel and do your best, including emotional awareness and stress management—to achieve your goals.

Maybe you have a particular goal or a healthful change you're trying to achieve that requires one or all of the following powers of your brain:

Impulse control
Emotional regulation
Comprehension
Critical thinking
Creativity
Empathy
Problem solving

All are powers of your prefrontal cortex, that we'll talk about much more.

But first, do you know WHY you want to achieve this particular goal or make this healthful change? In other words, what's your motivation to achieve it?

Without even realizing it, you may be relying on your unconscious stress response to keep you motivated—maybe anticipation of a reward, recognition, or acceptance. You may even be one of the millions of people who develop the unconscious habit of procrastination to trigger your unconscious stress response with that rush of adrenaline.

Maybe your stress comes from a fear of failure, rejection, or humiliation that motivates you to impress or attract someone, to feel liked, valued, or included. Or maybe your stress comes from your unconscious "fight or flight" response that motivates you to establish dominance and superiority, or seek vengeance to eliminate a perceived threat or enemy.

I ask not to make you feel bad, ashamed, guilty, or afraid, but rather to get your conscious mind thinking about the healthful outcomes you want to achieve and why, including how to maintain your motivation in the healthiest ways possible, even after you achieve this particular goal!

We all feel crappy at times—physically, mentally, emotionally, or a combination, since one affects the others in our interconnected neurological system (unless you're headless, in which case you're probably not reading or listening anyway).

The brain can also be a very sensitive subject, when our sense of identity—who we are and what we believe—are so closely related to what we think and feel.

Do you remember the last time you had a serious (or not-so-serious) discussion about brain health and function?

Maybe it's too stressful and confusing when there's still so much we don't know that we can't see or touch inside our bodies, and so much inside that we can't control. Maybe it's because the mystical and magical side of life is more fun when we don't look behind the curtain or learn how the sausage is made (spoiler alert… there's a person behind the curtain, and sausage is made of sausage).

Since the brain is something we can't see or control in any healthfully perfect way, and there's still so much we don't know, discussing brain function in itself can trigger an unconscious stress response since we tend to fear what we don't know, and what we can't control.

Human scholars and scientists have known about the basics of brain health and function for quite some time. Some evidence dates back to the earliest thinkers and philosophers around 200 B.C., but the field of Neuroscience is much more recent, and didn't become an official area of academic study until the 1960s.

When experts speak in terms that even the most intelligent of smart phones would find confusing, the brains of non-experts can get confused and overwhelmed, triggering an unconscious stress response just the same as a perceived threat (especially when it triggers a sense of shame). The brain naturally fights and resists against information it cannot comprehend or understand (that we call denial). In a way, it's our neurological resistance that gives our brain more time to process and determine fact from fiction, to come to terms with new information that may alter our perception of reality (that we call acceptance).

Unfortunately, when we don't discuss brain health and function, we leave ourselves more vulnerable to unhealthy mental influences, emotional abuses, and even malicious psychological attack, whether in the form of manipulative marketing, deceptive advertising, social media influencers, psychological grooming, brain washing, extremist recruiting, misinformation and disinformation, conspiracy theories, and political propaganda—that stress us out too.

Whether you enjoy being scared or not, we tend to ignore and avoid talking about brain health and function because it tends to scare us in some way. It's really a deeply sensitive and personal organ, as many of our organs tend to be. When was the last time you talked about digestive health or even sexual health at school or at work? Isn't it ironic for as much as we talk about human behaviors openly and often quite loudly and critically in public, discussing human organs and bodily functions seem practically taboo?

To which I say, "Poo."

When the information we are trying to share gets lost in translation and creates a defense response, then it completely defeats the purpose of communicating in the first place. We often refer to this phenomenon as "preaching to the choir" when we relay information in a way that only the people who already know, accept, and understand it can comprehend and process.

This is also why learning how to effectively communicate with those who don't already know, accept, or understand what you are trying to communicate has become a field of study in itself, in every language, as the study of Communications.

What can really give the brain a boost when communicating is including a bit of heart and humor that releases a bit of the neurochemical dopamine to reduce stress and increase a sense of safety and connection, optimizing critical thinking, problem solving, and comprehension. Understanding brain function is the real "secret" to know (with much more to come)!

Metaphors and analogies are also powerful tools when relaying information that's abstract or complex, by tapping into the existing neurological connections from what people already know—kind of like an on-ramp to understanding—thereby reducing the stress response and increasing memory and comprehension.

While this book may challenge your thinking and what you know so far, you will not be scolded, shamed, or put down for thinking, feeling, or behaving the way you do. To the contrary, I hope you feel enlightened, inspired, and encouraged as you learn more about your brain and body, and how you can feel and do your best amidst whatever challenges you face, which is what mental fitness is all about.

Efforts to change your behavior may seem like they're trying to change your sense of identity and who you are, by changing your beliefs, which is why the brain can be such a scary and difficult subject to discuss—by triggering an unconscious stress response that puts our defenses up, in "fight or flight" mode.

So I want to assure you that developing and maintaining healthful attitudes and behaviors is not a matter of changing your sense of self or identity, but rather a matter of awareness and understanding of your conscious and unconscious mind, to help you feel and do your best, to help you get where you want to go.

My aim is to provide valuable straight-forward information that you can use to better understand yourself (and others), to help you feel and do your best, to achieve whatever goals you have in life.

We'll discuss brain health and function in an easy-to-understand way, with a bit of heart and humor too, to energize and engage your brain in ways that allow you to comprehend, remember, and consider how mental fitness practices apply to your own brain health, fitness, and well-being (and I bet you thought I was just being silly).

Through it all, the ultimate aim is to empower you to seek the answers and support you need to achieve what YOU want to achieve.

MY BRAIN CAN'T POOP

1 WHAT IS FITNESS?

When you think of fitness, what comes to mind?

If your mind jumps to thoughts of physical fitness, don't feel bad. There's a reason "get in shape" has become synonymous, since physical shape is the concept of fitness most of us have been taught, told, and sold.

Whether it's due to our cultural obsession with physical strength and competition, sexual sexy sexiness, or our imbalanced healthcare system that focuses disproportionately on physical health (uh-hem), most of us immediately associate fitness with physical—with physical metrics, physical appearance, physical abilities, physical performance, physical size, shape, and weight—as well as what we physically consume and ingest.

What we unfortunately fail to realize in our obsession with the physical are the millions of bits of sensory information that we consume and ingest neurologically and physiologically, every second of every day, unconsciously in the brain, that influence every thought, feeling, behavior, and health outcome.

While physical fitness is absolutely important for your overall health, success, and well-being, it's also not the only aspect of fitness (or dare I say, even the most important).

Since your brain is what drives your body, fitness really has less to do with specific physical abilities and everything to do with mental abilities (just ask any Paralympic athlete!).

This goes for every person, of every age, race, and gender, without exception.

If we were to shift just a fraction of the hundreds of billions of dollars we collectively spend on physical fitness in the U.S. alone each year, to invest in brain health efforts that make mental fitness a priority, imagine what a difference we could make in identifying, managing, healing, and preventing many of the ills that ail us.

While making a societal shift to flip fitness on its head is a bit like trying to turn the Titanic, you can absolutely take charge of your own life by securing your own life preserver. You can take charge of your own ship by making your own brain health and mental fitness a priority. When you become the captain of your own health and fitness, you also become a powerful influence for others by setting a healthful example, empowering them to prioritize their own brain health and mental fitness too (that can help us avoid hitting that nasty iceberg in the first place).

You can choose to prioritize and invest in your own mental fitness as much (or more) as you prioritize and invest in your physical fitness. It will require a critical mass to make a real change in our educational, political, and healthcare systems— but just as every step counts toward achieving your goals, so does every person count in making this societal shift, including YOU!

The relationship between mental health and mental fitness is similar to the relationship between physical health and physical fitness. Though health and fitness are related, they are different and should not be confused.

There are many interpretations of health and fitness, so for purposes of this discussion, the word "health" generally refers to the state of being free from illness or injury, or the "healthful" steps and practices to take in preventing or healing from an illness or injury that may require medical care or therapy.

The term "fitness" generally relates to your ability to adapt and thrive in your environment. Fitness is your preparedness or ability to achieve a specific goal, including the goal of living your best life possible. You can still be "fit" to adapt, thrive, achieve, and live your best life possible even when you have a health condition, illness, injury, imbalance, or impairment that affects your specific fitness practice, that may differ from others (at the discretion of your healthcare provider, of course).

Just like physical fitness, mental fitness is never one-and-done either, and requires continual practice.

Even when you are otherwise "healthy," you may not be "fit" to achieve a certain goal without proper training or practice. Likewise, you may be fit to perform and achieve a certain goal even when you have other health issues or challenges.

Understanding health and fitness in this way is absolutely essential for purposes of maintaining motivation and inclusion, to believe in your abilities even when you're not feeling your best—when your best can change from day-to-day, month-to-month, and year-to-year.

The point being, do NOT let the state of your health discourage you from working toward your fitness goals!

3

Mental fitness is all about empowering you with the information, practices, and support you need to thrive in your environment, to feel and do your best, to achieve your goals— regardless of physical shape, appearance, or abilities.

Whatever your physical abilities, prioritizing your mental fitness as a critical component of your brain health is an important first step toward achievement and well-being. By focusing on brain health, you can help eliminate the fear, shame, and stigma that so often get in the way of finding, delivering, and receiving the care people need to achieve healthful outcomes, that must include healthful thoughts, feelings, and behaviors influenced by healthy information, understanding, and support.

Whether physical or mental, fitness practices are never a substitute for physical or mental healthcare, but are an important supplement to optimize your health and well-being. Just as you would with any physical symptoms, it's critical to be aware of mental and emotional symptoms, and have them checked by a healthcare professional.

While physical and mental healthcare services are most often provided by a licensed medical doctor or clinician in a hospital or clinical setting, physical and mental fitness services are often guided by a fitness instructor, coach, or trainer—whether outdoors, at work, at home, or at a fitness center.

Fitness practices proactively help you improve or maintain your mental and physical health, performance, and well-being by making the most of the abilities you have—to help you adapt and develop, or even heal and recover (at the discretion of your healthcare provider, of course). Maintaining your health and well-being is a continual process of nourishing and healing, especially when dealing with an illness, injury, or imbalance.

Mental fitness practices focus on raising awareness of the various mental, physical, and emotional signals to help you better understand and care for your brain and body, to navigate the ups and downs of life in healthful ways, including seeking proper care and support. Just ask any body builder how important it is to ask for a spotter when they're lifting a heavy load, and they'll tell you how important it is to both prevent injury and increase motivation. The same goes for any heavy mental or emotional load you're carrying too.

2 FOCUS ON BRAIN FUNCTION

To truly thrive, it's important to care for your mind as a critical function of your brain—as a neurological and physiological part of your body, made up of billions of neurons and neuropathways that get turned on and off by hundreds of neurochemicals.

Fitness really begins with how you think and feel; that is, how you process your thoughts and feelings. Even when you consciously know the healthful actions to take to succeed and stay healthy, it's ultimately how you think and feel about it that determines your success or failure, influencing the choices you make and the actions you take (or don't).

Mental fitness practices can be used to support:

1. Personal achievement and well-being
2. Diversity, equity, and inclusion (i.e., community achievement and well-being)
3. Change management (i.e., adaptation and de-escalation)
4. Optimization of healthful influences (i.e., social, environmental, nutritional, and chemical influences)

When it comes to fitness practices that help you feel and do your best, often just getting started and staying motivated are the hardest parts. Even when you know that you can do the fitness exercises and practices, you may struggle with limiting thoughts and feelings that tap your energy and hold you back. Maybe it's something you were told or experienced at some point in life that got electrochemically forged into your long-term memory deep in your unconscious mind (the neurology of which we'll talk more about in a bit).

These deeply embedded thoughts and feelings are not easy to consciously change or simply shake off when they get repeated and reinforced neurologically, over and over again in your head, whether by your own rumination (that may be associated with anxiety or depression), by your environment that constantly triggers those thoughts and feelings (possibly even an unkempt space that reflects the lack of care you feel about yourself), or by others around you who either intentionally or unintentionally reinforce those limiting thoughts and feelings that can become part of your identity, how you perceive yourself, and how others perceive you (a sort of self-perpetuating cycle that repeats and reinforces itself).

Very often we may unconsciously seek negative attention and experiences when we feel negatively about ourselves, as a kind of confirmation bias that reinforces how we already think and feel about ourselves, even when those thoughts and feelings are toxic and unhealthy (that's sometimes referred to as "self-sabotage"). By lowering expectations, we relieve the stress we put on ourselves and others to think or feel differently, to soothe our own unconscious stress response.

It might sound irrational to say that our own brain does not want to change for our own health and well-being, but that's just how our unconscious stress response works sometimes. When challenging our thoughts and feelings becomes stressful, our unconscious stress response gets energized that takes energy away from our prefrontal cortex that requires conscious effort to redirect energy from our amygdala to our prefrontal cortex.

Forging healthy neuropathways would be challenging enough without those limiting thoughts and feelings that cause mental and emotional resistance, and direct energy to the amygdala instead of the prefrontal cortex, much like trying to redirect a raging river when you can't hold the water back. The water (or neurological signals) will continue to flow down the path of least resistance (that is the existing pathway where it will always hit the amygdala first) until another pathway is forged to help redirect the flow, by reducing resistance, and allowing the old pathway to dry up and become weaker.

Developing healthier habits and routines—including healthier thought patterns and stress management techniques—takes time, conscious effort, reinforcement, and repetition to develop and maintain those healthful neuropathways, thoughts, and feelings that you need to succeed and achieve your goals.

Just like your muscles and other functional organs in your body, your brain needs to be properly prepared and warmed-up before doing intense work—to get blood and neurochemicals flowing in an optimal way, to either forge or reinforce those healthful pathways. Putting stress on our neurological and physiological system before your brain is prepared and engaged in a healthful way can result in experiences like brain fog, irritability, or confusion. This is the importance of a progressive approach that prepares the brain and body for work in a healthful way, starting with the foundational elements of your system on which everything else can grow and develop.

I created the 4D Fit Mental Fitness Model℠ as an easy-to-understand framework that offers a variety of progressive mental fitness practices, including the importance of self-awareness, sleep, grief, forgiveness, creativity, nutrition, hydration, social connection, breathing, and movement, that focus on developing the foundation of your neurological and physiological system:

Level 1: Balance (awareness)

Level 2: Flexibility (processing)

Level 3: Rest & Recovery (self-care)

Level 4: Strength & Endurance (maintenance & motivation)

Mental fitness practices focus on how you process your thoughts and feelings to understand how your brain and body work together.

By focusing on mental fitness, you will be better able to identify what influences your emotions, and what drives your conscious and unconscious mind as functional areas of your brain, including your thoughts, feelings, and behaviors.

Much like how you first learn to stay afloat in the water before learning how to swim, mental fitness practices promote brain health incrementally by focusing on emotional awareness, processing, and self-care practices to help you navigate the ups and downs in life by prioritizing your brain health and mental well-being, to feel and do your best, to get where you want to go.

Mental fitness—in terms of optimizing performance and well-being—is a relatively new concept in the wellness arena that promotes the healthful thoughts and feelings that lead to healthful behaviors, neurologically and physiologically.

The focus on mental fitness has been gaining traction in recent years largely due to increasing rates of physical and mental health conditions associated with chronic stress and elevated levels of cortisol—including heart disease, obesity, cancer, anxiety, depression, eating disorders, violence and aggressions (including physical, sexual, and emotional abuse), drug abuse, and suicide—that are also compounded by the effects of shame and stigma around mental, emotional, and behavioral health that get in the way of finding and providing treatment, healing, and preventive care.

Mental fitness is all about understanding the basics of brain health and function so you can apply what you know to your daily life in simple and practical ways. Increasing awareness of what you think and how you feel, as well as what influences your thoughts, feelings, and behaviors, can help you decide and find what you need to feel and do your best. The aim of mental fitness is not to control what you think and feel, but to embrace, explore, and understand yourself better, to inspire more questions, ideas, and considerations as you navigate life.

Mental fitness practices focus on learning and development to help you take those important first steps to feel and do your best, including emotional awareness, stress management, meditation, creativity, controlled breathing, better sleep, nutrition, and physical exercise, or even the help of a licensed clinical counselor or therapist who can provide the care you need beyond what fitness practices can provide.

So why don't we teach basic brain health and function at school, work, and in every gym and doctor's office?

It might seem obvious to say that behavior is the result of mental and emotional processes, that involve neurological repetition, reward, and reinforcement, yet in all of my academic and professional experience—in psychology, marketing, fitness, mental health, political activism, and D.E.I.—rarely (if ever) has brain health or brain function been considered a priority.

I have my theories—whether due to basic human fears and the short-lived bliss we find in ignorance, how it's easier to blame someone else than take responsibility ourselves, how powers of influence work best when we are unaware of them, or how we finance (and insure) our fragmented healthcare system, or all of the above (or something else that I am totally unaware of). Your guess is really as good as mine.

What we do know is the U.S. spends hundreds of billions of dollars each year on marketing and advertising to influence behaviors, as our health crises continue to rise. The paradox being that while we are exposed to vast amounts of unhealthful influences—in what we hear, read, watch, buy, click, follow, drink, and eat—that all want us to choose and consume, regardless of the health impact on ourselves or others, we still expect healthful results.

Is it because we don't teach or understand how the human brain operates? Is it because we believe the magic of "willpower" should be stronger than our neurology and physiology?

Whatever the reason we have historically failed to acknowledge and teach brain health and function, the most important part of mental fitness is awareness—awareness of brain health and function, including healthful influences and practices you can use to support your own brain health and mental well-being, neurologically and physiologically, even when our educational, political, and healthcare systems have a long way to go to meet the basic needs of every human brain.

This is about as political as I get since politics can be an unhealthful influence in itself, pitting people against people for the purpose of power and control.

To which I again say, "Poo."

It might seem like a "no brainer" to say your brain is the most important organ in your body, yet it's often the most abused, neglected, and misunderstood organ as well.

When it comes to improving your overall fitness, we often limit the concept of fitness to just physical, focusing on what we can see and measure in three dimensions—being the visible body, including biometrics and behaviors. Therefore, what we can't see gets ignored—like our mind, senses, and emotions— that are electro-chemical processes that involve physical organs, cells, and tissue as well, including your brain, neurons, hormones, and neurotransmitters.

While we can easily observe and measure physical outcomes, behaviors, and appearances, the mental processes behind attitudes and behaviors are much harder to observe—hidden in the brain.

Of course every part of you is incredibly important to your health and well-being, so no disrespect to your other awesome organs or the life-giving energy that runs through you— whether you consider that energy your spirit, soul, essence, or not (that we'll talk more about later, and why I leave the topic of spirituality up to you).

Your brain is the most important organ in your body quite simply because it's connected to every part of your body in ways that your other organs are not. Your brain consists of billions of neurons (tiny cells that send and receive signals throughout your body by using electric and chemical signals— otherwise known as electrochemical) and hundreds of neurochemicals (the chemicals that interact with your neurons to turn those electric signals on or off). It's these neurochemical signals shooting out of and into your brain that influence every thought, feeling, behavior, and body function.

And like every other part of your body, your brain requires

proper care, nutrition, and development to meet the ever-changing demands of life.

In many ways, your brain is what defines who you are as a unique human individual, in how you process, perceive, interact, and navigate the natural world around you, including how you perceive and identify yourself as an individual (even when you're an identical twin!).

You don't have a second brain as a back-up, nor can your brain be replaced or transplanted by another brain or mechanical simulator (at least not yet). Your brain continues to operate unconsciously even when you're not conscious, or other parts of your body may be impaired due to genetic difference, illness, or injury. As long as your brain is alive, so are you.

As painfully challenging as adapting to a physical impairment, injury, illness, or imbalance can be, you can absolutely continue to thrive as a viable member of society, thanks to your amazing human brain.

(I told you that you are amazing!)

Your amazingness can also be mind-blowing and even a bit scary to think about. With so many moving parts and pieces happening invisibly inside of you at the cellular level all at once, all of the time, when you're asleep and awake, you start to realize how little you actually have conscious control over most of the time, and how much happens without your conscious awareness.

Trying to understand your extremely complex human brain can be quite overwhelming and stressful to think about, especially when you don't know where to start.

As humans, we tend to fear what we can't see, understand, or control, that can trigger a stress response that leads to anxiety, worry, and concern. When so much remains a mystery beyond our comprehension, we can quickly jump to conclusions that add to the toxic shame, stress, and stigma.

Ignorance might be bliss to a point, when we reduce stress by ignoring something and not thinking or worrying about it; but when we fail to consider and understand something, we also put ourselves at greater risk of unhealthy decisions, behaviors, and mistakes, that can lead to illness, injury, or worse.

This is also why knowledge is power—so long as you know how to manage your stress and worry to use it in a healthful way (to not just stress, worry, or fight about it).

So fear not, fellow human.

The good news is that as challenging and stressful as learning about your brain might be, discussing brain health and function in a simple, practical, and non-judgmental way can help reduce stress by approaching thoughts, feelings, and behaviors as a matter of neurochemical function of your very human brain that needs proper care to optimize performance.

One way to simplify your neurological system is to think of your body as the vehicle and your brain as the driver.

Whether you're a gearhead or not (like me), you likely know that proper care and maintenance is important to optimize performance, to keep the vehicle running smoothly for as long as possible.

It is also the responsibility of the driver to ensure sufficient training, understanding, maintenance, and operation. (I learned this the hard way when the engine blew up in my first car, after I forgot to get the oil changed… that was one expensive WOOPS!)

Of course the best way to ensure driver's safety is through education, to learn how to drive safely and maintain your vehicle. Driving recklessly or not maintaining your vehicle put both car and driver at risk, as well as the other cars and drivers on the road.

Similarly, it is the function of your brain to operate, navigate, and maintain your body to ensure your health, safety, and well-being; and just as the driver requires proper training to drive and maintain the vehicle, so does your brain. We need to know how to fill the tank with proper fuel, and how or where to take our vehicle for proper maintenance and repairs, to run as long as possible, to get where we want to go.

When it comes to the human brain and body, we very often put in unhealthy fuel and operate under the influence of toxic chemicals that put wear and tear on our internal systems, and cause serious harm and long-term complications with operations.

While your brain may be the most important part of your vehicle, when it comes to basic health, fitness, and well-being, we often focus on what we can see, and forget to look under the hood, when everything below the neck (the vehicle) is being driven by everything above the neck (your head).

And like the rest of your body, your brain requires proper care, rest, nourishment, healing, and exercise to healthfully drive your thoughts, feelings, and behaviors that directly impact your overall health, fitness, and success.

What you can do is find a good pit crew (whether trainers, instructors, doctors, or therapists) to help you learn how to operate and maintain your vehicle. Even the best doctors, therapists, trainers, and instructors cannot do the work for you, just as the best medicines and treatments only work as well as your brain and body can heal and process them.

The only person who can actually heal, grow, and develop your brain and body is YOU. Others can help guide and support you by providing information and access to necessary treatments, medicines, or nutrients, but the actual biological work and neurochemical energy that is required for you to heal, grow, and develop comes from inside of your living and breathing human brain and body.

When we limit the concept of fitness to only things we can physically observe, we tend to ignore the role of the brain, thereby limiting our full potential.

Mental health isn't just about illness, injury, imbalance, or impairment either, but how you manage and maintain your mental well-being as part of a mental fitness practice.

Unfortunately, the term "fitness" has been monopolized by the physical fitness industry, when "fitness" is really about your ability to perform and thrive in your environment, to achieve the goals you want to achieve, which has less to do with your physical abilities and everything to do with your mental abilities.

Fitness is about feeling your best to do your best, with the abilities you have, whatever they might be—to comprehend and think critically, to regulate emotions and impulses, to manage stress, to navigate problems and challenges in healthful ways, to achieve and accomplish your goals, while maintaining your motivation along the way.

The purpose of health and fitness really is not about expecting people (or the world) to be perfect, that is a subjective term in itself since what is "perfect" for you is likely different than what is "perfect" for me—influenced by our neurology and physiology that influence our needs and desires. What is important is to understand what influences us as human beings, as fellow navigators of life, as essential parts of nature and our environment, so we can increase the healthful and reduce the unhealthful, to navigate life as best we can, for as long as we can.

We'll explore what influences your brain health and function inside and out, and why—from the food you eat to the friends you keep, to activities you do and the information you consume—that affect your well-being, including how you think and feel, especially when you're trying to develop healthier habits and behaviors.

While we'll mainly focus on the brain, it's also important to understand how your brain health relates to the rest of your body, including your gut health, metabolism, and digestion, through the exchange of very important neurological and physiological signals. This is often why we say "trust your gut," since your brain receives signals from your gut faster than your conscious mind can process them.

Similar to your gut health, what you consume through your senses—including your vision, hearing, taste, smell, touch, and internal sensations—influence your brain health and function neurologically and physiologically as much as what you physically ingest influences your gut health and function.

Since your brain can't poop, however, there are other processes that your brain and body go through to relieve the neurological stress and neurochemical waste that build up in your brain and body too.

Just like digestion, it's more healthful to let out the neurological and neurochemical byproduct of your mental processes (that we experience as thoughts and feelings) in a healthful way, rather than holding it all in (preferably without dumping our toxic waste on someone else).

Self-expression is a lot like fiber in that talking, journaling, or even artistic expression can help you process thoughts and feelings that are otherwise just abstract neurological signals firing in your brain, until you let them out through your words or other form of emotional expression, like relieving mental and emotional constipation.

Sleep is also a critical part of your health and well-being, for the neurological processes your brain and body go through during critical sleep cycles to relax your system, prune old neurological synapses, and flush toxic physiological byproducts that accumulate during the day. One such byproduct is the neurochemical adenosine that builds up in your system from regular cellular growth and activity during the day, that build up to make you tired at the end of the day.

Caffeine actually works by directly blocking the tiring effects of adenosine in your brain, thereby preventing you from feeling tired, and feeling more awake. In small doses, caffeine may have a healthful effect by stimulating your neurological system.

However, this neurochemical effect is also why you might experience a caffeine crash when you artificially keep yourself awake with caffeine, without allowing your brain and body the proper sleep you need to naturally flush the adenosine from your system. When the caffeine finally wears off (or you develop an adaptive resistance to it), whatever amount of adenosine is left in your system comes rushing back, altering your body chemistry in a way that can make you incredibly tired and cranky.

Those with more sensitive neurological systems may be extra sensitive to the effects of caffeine as well, that can make sleeping more difficult and even trigger symptoms of anxiety (that might also depend on the type and quality of caffeine being consumed).

Speaking of sleep, dreaming is a lot like passing gas, as you might both rumble and mumble. While this might give you a chuckle (or repulse you completely), dreams really are a byproduct of your mental activity. They are the neurological residue of your thoughts, feelings, and stress that neurologically build up in your unconscious mind, much like gas builds up as you digest. This build-up needs a way to be processed and released, which happens as you sleep. This is also why some dreams might be more pleasant than others (dare I say less stinky), depending on what your brain consumed that day.

Mindfulness and meditation, on the other hand, are a lot like an antacid for your brain, in how they can help calm your mind and emotions, neurologically and physiologically as well.

This not only applies to you, but each and every human being.

3 YOUR CONSCIOUS AND UNCONSCIOUS MIND

When it comes to maintaining your brain health and mental fitness, it's important to know the basics. There are both conscious and unconscious functions in your brain that control mental, emotional, and behavioral functions, as well as every other bodily function (even when you're asleep!).

The powers of your brain and body are absolutely mind blowing, especially since 90 percent of your brain function happens unconsciously—without you even thinking about it. Your brain and body are constantly working unconsciously to achieve homeostasis (that's why you poop, to rebalance your system too). You don't have to consciously think about it or tell your body to digest and get rid of the waste—it just does.

Some of these amazing functions work simultaneously, like how your heart and lungs work together to distribute oxygenated blood throughout your body. Others work opposite each other, like your sympathetic and parasympathetic nervous systems—which is why you can either be stressed (with an activate sympathetic nervous system) or you can be relaxed (with an active parasympathetic nervous system), but you cannot be both stressed and relaxed at the very same time, due to how your nervous system works.

When there's a sudden change or imbalance in your system—such as an infection or injury—neurochemical signals fire that result in physical, emotional, and even behavioral symptoms as your brain and body respond to the infection or injury. You might experience neurological symptoms like pain, dizziness, or instability, or even swelling and inflammation, as your immune system kicks in to try to correct whatever is causing the imbalance—even if the cause of the imbalance is your own neurological or physiological system (in the case of an allergy or autoimmune disorder).

This is similar to the way your brain experiences change and grief as well. When there is a sudden neurological or physiological shift or imbalance, your brain and body are forced to adapt and adjust, that can result in physical, emotional, and even behavioral symptoms when the shift or imbalance becomes too uncomfortable or painful.

The major difference being that while we can physically see or otherwise observe a physical change, trauma, or imbalance (like a broken leg), we cannot see mental and emotional changes, traumas, or imbalances (like depression), and therefore tend to overlook and underestimate mental and emotional change, trauma, and imbalance as less critical or significant.

Your mental system is one of the many neurological and physiological functions going on in your body at every moment of every day without much conscious effort. So you may or may not be surprised to know that your brain and body already unconsciously do most of the mental fitness practices we'll talk about—like breathing, moving your body, drinking, eating, talking, looking, listening, feeling, sleeping, dreaming, and laughing—most of which you practically do automatically without much conscious thought or effort.

Just as your gut has digestive processes to absorb and make use of what you physically consume, your brain also has mental processes to absorb and make use of what you consume mentally through your sensory organs. Similar to how your gut health and digestive system are influenced by different internal and external factors—like what, when, and how you eat—so are your brain health and mental processes influenced by different internal and external factors as well—including what, when, and how you consume sensory information, including sights, sounds, tastes, smells, touch, vibrations, and other sensations.

If your brain operated more like your gut, you could extract the healthful bits of information and experiences, and poop out the stuff that doesn't do you any good—that just builds up as toxic waste in your system and makes you feel ill.

While your mental system doesn't work exactly like your digestive system, your brain does detoxify and rebalance in neurological and physiological ways too. To some extent, you can also improve and develop how your mental system works neurologically and physiologically with proper education, care, and exercise, to support your brain health and mental well-being (that also includes improving your gut health!).

It's easy to practice healthful habits when life is easy, but is extra difficult when life gets hard. It's not for lack of willpower, or lack of desire. There's a neurological reason why one of the greatest challenges we face is maintaining our own motivation to maintain our health and well-being.

We often know what we "should" do, but have a hard time doing it, in large part because we've been conditioned in these modern consumer-driven times to crave instant gratification and immediate results. When we are overly stressed, we may not even believe that making an effort will make a difference or be worthwhile (since we wanted it yesterday).

It's not so much a matter of "what" you think but "how" you think, how you process your thoughts and feelings, how to be aware of what is influencing your thoughts, feelings, and behaviors in healthful or unhealthful ways, so you can reduce the internal effects of stress, to take better care of your brain and maintain your motivation.

Mental fitness focuses on practices that empower you to proactively balance your unconscious stress response in a healthfully conscious way—to navigate the stresses and challenges of life, so you can feel and do your best, to achieve your goals.

While we've come a long way since the last ice pick lobotomy was performed (and killed the patient) in the 1960s, we're still not taught how to care for our brains and mental health as much as we're taught how to care for our bodies and physical health.

We would never shame or tell someone who was exhibiting symptoms of an undiagnosed physical health condition to "shake it off," and would likely recommend immediate medical attention; but we are often quick to shame someone who is exhibiting symptoms of an undiagnosed mental health condition.

Similar to physical health, caring for your mental health takes conscious effort. It requires identifying and seeking healthful influences, and reducing or avoiding unhealthful influences, to balance your neurological and physiological system, to optimize your health, performance, and well-being. Your brain and body respond to internal and external influences, including thoughts and feelings that are unconscious neurological and physiological responses, especially when you are stressed.

And there are a lot of stressors in life.

When we feel stressed and don't feel safe, our unconscious stress response kicks in to protect us, much like our unconscious immune response. When we are in a stressed state, we are emotionally vulnerable, since it is our amygdala that is in control and driving our unconscious thoughts and feelings. The stress response of fear can especially inhibit critical thinking, emotional regulation, and impulse control (all powered by the prefrontal cortex), which is why fear is so effective at persuading and influencing our thoughts, feelings, and behaviors, often in unhealthy ways.

Preventive mental fitness practices promote emotional awareness and stress management to navigate change, grief, and the challenges of life in healthful ways. An ounce of prevention is definitely worth a pound of cure when we're talking about brain health that influences every thought, idea, decision, and action we take (or don't).

With so many moving parts and pieces to brain function, the main parts of the brain we'll focus on are your *amygdala* (that powers your unconscious mind and stress response) and your *prefrontal cortex* (that powers your conscious higher-functioning mind).

The complex neurological activity between your amygdala and prefrontal cortex impacts your mental health and well-being in significant ways. These two parts of your brain essentially compete for energy and attention. This is why mental fitness focuses on practices to help calm the amygdala and engage the prefrontal cortex, to optimize and strengthen healthful brain function to build resilience.

Your hot-headed amygdala

First, let's get to know your *amygdala*. Your amygdala is the most primitive part of your brain that powers your unconscious stress response, and is fully formed at birth.

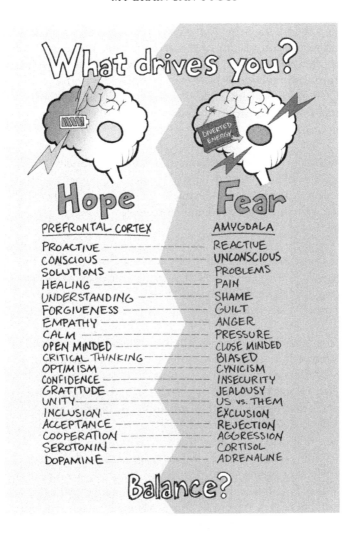

It's a small almond-shaped area connected to long-term memory that receives neurological signals first to sense, remember, and react to danger (e.g., kicking, crying, screaming, etc.) before you even learn to walk, talk, or defend yourself.

Interestingly, since your amygdala has a similar size and shape to an almond, the name "amygdala" actually comes from the Latin word "amygdalum" that means almond. The amygdala is also often referred to as your "lizard brain" since it's so similar in form and function as the brains of other less-evolved animals like lizards (that does not mean you are part lizard, unless you're from a galaxy far-far-away … in which case, nanoo nanoo!).

I personally like to call the amygdala your "baby brain" since it is responsible for those defensive temperamental behaviors we associate with children and babies—the screaming and crying when we're hungry, scared, uncomfortable, or otherwise want something.

Due to the progressive way your brain and body develop, the amygdala is also one of the last parts of your brain to deteriorate, especially associated with neurodegenerative diseases like dementia.

Your amygdala is part of your limbic system that is involved in emotional and behavioral responses, especially related to basic survival instincts like feeding, sex, and physical protection. It is directly connected to your *autonomic nervous system* (ANS) that controls your glands, organs, and automatic physiological functions. This is why your amygdala receives neurological signals first, and reacts unconsciously, before the higher-functioning conscious part of your brain receives the signals (namely your prefrontal cortex that we'll talk about next). It's also directly connected to your long-term memory, which is why it's so easy to remember those exciting or even traumatic experiences, when your stress and emotions are heightened.

If you've ever seen illustrations of your nervous system, it really looks like a plant, with tiny branches that spread all through your brain and body, carrying electrical signals from one branch to another—known as neurons. The neurons are turned on and off by hundreds of different neurochemicals.

For purposes of mental fitness, it's not as important to know the names of all the different parts and pieces as it is to be aware of all the work that your nervous system is doing inside your brain and body.

Your autonomic nervous system is also divided into two branches. One is your *parasympathetic nervous system* that carries electrochemical signals involved with rest, repair, and digestion. The other is your *sympathetic nervous system* that carries signals involved with stress, and helps divert needed blood and energy away from those organs to your heart, lungs, and muscles instead, increasing your heart rate and breathing rate, to prepare your body for physical activity. This unconscious stress response is often referred to as your "fight or flight" response. Sometimes "freeze" is a response, when your stress response overloads your system in such a way that your brain can't process how to react or respond, and practically shuts down—a sort of momentary paralysis.

Your amygdala is connected to your autonomic (unconscious) nervous system, and triggers your stress response that diverts energy to the sympathetic branch of your nervous system. When your amygdala is relaxed, your parasympathetic nervous system is activated.

This is why it's so hard to sleep and relax when you're stressed, and why your digestion, metabolism, hormone levels, and even your immune system are compromised when you are in a stressed state. It's all a result of your amygdala that triggers your sympathetic nervous system and pumps the stress hormone *cortisol* into your system.

Beyond healthful habits and behaviors, cortisol also impacts your physical health in significant ways, contributing to everything from skin conditions to heart disease, from mood disorders to obesity.

As your front-line defense, your amygdala does not like being wrong, and for very good reason. You depend on your amygdala to sense danger, to take action against threats, to stay alive. This is why your stress response might also cause confirmation bias in your unconscious attempt to prove your amygdala right, to reinforce what you perceive mentally as a threat is in fact a real physical threat.

Your long-term memory kicks in to remember those threats, so you are better prepared and able to identify, prevent, or avoid them next time. This is why your unconscious stress response can also result in unconscious biases when someone or something resembles a perceived threat, or even an emotional preference or sense of safety (such as that sense of safety we feel around friends or family).

Being motivated by problems, threats, and stress can contribute to a toxic level of cortisol in your system that can also contribute to toxic attitudes and behaviors, including toxic relationships and eating habits. Reducing the toxic effects of stress requires tremendous care and effort to calm the unconscious stress response of the amygdala to fully engage the prefrontal cortex and rebalance your neurochemical system. Very often clinical counseling and therapy are needed to heal the neuropathways that have been forged through repeated traumatic experiences that reinforce those neuropathways, making them extremely difficult to heal and adjust if even painful, as the amygdala may respond even more severely, perceiving the healing attempt as a threat in itself. This is why we can never heal someone who does not want to heal, who finds motivation in their pain and stress, who finds it too challenging to engage their prefrontal cortex.

While we may require help and support, and try to help and support others, we can really only ever truly heal ourselves, that may include seeking, finding, and accepting help and support.

Your unconscious stress response is not something to be ashamed of, but to be aware of. Unconscious functions include breathing and digestion, and even movements and behaviors that you have done so many times over and over again (through repetition and reinforcement) that you no longer need to consciously think about them (a.k.a. muscle memory). Some forms of muscle memory include walking, talking, and even driving, since you can do these things with little conscious effort or attention (for better or worse, when we might automatically do or say something without consciously thinking first).

This is why you might do things "mindlessly" or even be called "hot-headed" when you are stressed—when you're being unconsciously driven by emotions triggered by your amygdala. Sometimes your response results in a healthful form of self-defense, that motivates you to fight or flee, to seek shelter, safety, or what you need; while other times your response may result in unhealthful outcomes, when your overwhelming desire for instant gratification to soothe your stress response contributes to impulsive, unwise, harmful, or otherwise unhealthy behaviors or decisions.

This is why the practices of "mindfulness" is so important to mental fitness, to be consciously aware of those thoughts and feelings triggered by your unconscious stress response that can influence your decisions and behaviors—that requires conscious effort to engage your prefrontal cortex.

Your cool-headed prefrontal cortex

Next, let's get to know the higher-functioning conscious part of your brain, your *prefrontal cortex*. This is the part of your brain that mental fitness practices really aim to engage and develop, since it requires conscious effort like a muscle.

Your prefrontal cortex is the most evolved or highest-functioning part of your brain connected to short-term working memory that powers conscious executive functions—including comprehension, critical thinking, problem solving, creativity, empathy, impulse control, and emotional regulation.

Your prefrontal cortex makes up the outer layer of your brain with billions of neurons packed together so tightly that it gives your brain a grayish color, that's often referred to as "gray matter." As you grow, learn, and develop, more neurons form, and rather than your whole head increasing in size until you can no longer wear a hat or fit through a doorway, the general size and shape remains the same while your gray matter folds in on itself to create more surface area, like crunching more and more fabric into a container, giving your brain that wrinkly appearance.

Your prefrontal cortex continues to grow and develop until it's fully matured around the age of twenty-five.

When our prefrontal cortex is underdeveloped, impaired, or inhibited, or the amygdala becomes traumatized or overactive, our unconscious stress response becomes harder to regulate.

This imbalance may result in symptoms associated with various mental, emotional, and behavioral health conditions, neurological disorders, and even cognitive differences that often overlap.

We often classify behaviors as "acting like a child" or "acting immature" when we have limited emotional regulation and impulse control, when our amygdala is more active and developed than our prefrontal cortex, especially when the prefrontal cortex is impaired or underdeveloped.

Since your prefrontal cortex is the last part of your brain to develop, it is also the last part of your brain to receive neurological signals through your nervous system that are first sent to your amygdala as your unconscious defense center, thereby taking energy away from your prefrontal cortex when your amygdala gets triggered. This is why it takes conscious effort and practice to be consciously aware of your emotions and stress triggers, in order to redirect energy to your conscious brain, to regulate your unconscious stress response.

Since the prefrontal cortex is the last part of the brain to develop, it is also the most susceptible to developmental disorders such as Fetal Alcohol Spectrum Disorders—that can occur when a fetus is exposed to any level of alcohol at any time during pregnancy.

As previously explained with the amygdala, due to the progressive way your brain and body develop, the prefrontal cortex is also the first area to show signs of deterioration from degenerative diseases like dementia, with the loss of short-term memory and impaired executive functioning being some of the first signs and symptoms.

People on the Autism Spectrum also have differences in the way their prefrontal cortex operates, that can result in challenges with managing stress, navigating change, regulating emotions, controlling impulses, or feeling empathy (to be understood as a fact of neurodiversity, and not a moral deficiency).

What if we understood that every human brain is as diverse as every human body?

What if we no longer expected people to think, feel, and behave in the same ways, and instead make efforts to understand and support their individual brain health and function?

What would it mean for our systems of education, healthcare, business, employment, entertainment, justice, media, marketing, religion, law enforcement, politics, and even the military?

What would it mean for treating and preventing unhealthy thoughts, feelings, and behaviors that contribute to mental abuse, physical abuse, sexual abuse, chemical abuse, eating disorders, trauma, heart disease, cancer, obesity, depression, anxiety, and suicide?

What would it mean for empowering people to understand themselves and each other, to feel and do their best, to foster a more healthful community?

4 NEURODIVERSITY

Just as no two bodies are exactly the same, neither are any two brains.

While your genetics, abilities, environment, education, experience, beliefs, and identity are all as unique as you are, the basic functions of the human brain apply to all—including the unconscious stress response of the amygdala, and the higher functioning consciousness of the prefrontal cortex. As humans, we are all similar in this way. Not to say that all human brains develop or operate exactly the same, any more than every human body develops and operates exactly the same. Understanding the similarities and differences in our neurology and physiology is so critical for individual care, healing, and well-being, when one size rarely fits all—that is the importance of neurodiversity.

When it comes to understanding the cognitive, mental, emotional, perceptual, experiential, and behavioral differences among people, it's important to understand neurological differences in the brain, and the many variables that influence brain health, function, and development—without shame or judgment.

As we learn more and more about the brain, the concept of neurodiversity is becoming increasingly important—to help raise awareness about the variations in brain function and development that drive different learning styles, abilities, emotions, and behaviors. It's also important to understand the impact of stress on your brain and the importance of stress management, to optimize executive functions of the prefrontal cortex, that could be significantly impacted by a neurological, mental health, or other physiological condition.

Understanding how your brain operates is probably the most important step you can take toward feeling and doing your best to achieve your goals, and knowing what and why things influence you the way they do. With greater knowledge and awareness, we are better able to understand and manage stressors that impact our thoughts, feelings, and behaviors in healthier ways, to avoid shaming, punishing, and further traumatizing individuals who have likely already been shamed, punished, and traumatized for their thoughts, feelings, and behaviors, who need proper care, treatment, and healing instead.

When we acknowledge and accept how a brain that has developed differently, or is not yet fully developed, is going to think, feel, and act as such, then we are better able to comprehend and understand what drives healthful behaviors, and how to influence diverse brains in diversely healthful ways.

It's often the prefrontal cortex that is most impacted, making the unconscious stress response of the amygdala more powerful and pronounced, and more challenging to manage. This imbalance can further inhibit mental functions that we so often take for granted as "normal" or "mature," and tend to shame as "abnormal" or "immature" thoughts, feelings, or behaviors, when our emotional regulation and impulse control is inhibited or impaired by our unconscious stress response.

The topic of neurodiversity often focuses on developmental differences among people on the Autism spectrum, or differences among people born with a Fetal Alcohol Spectrum Disorder (FASD), but neurodiversity really applies to everyone on the broader spectrum of diverse neurological functioning and development across individuals. It's important to be aware of these differences and variations in neurological development and abilities to better understand ourselves and each other, how we often think, feel, learn, comprehend, perceive, believe, and behave differently.

Raising awareness about neurodiversity helps reduce fear, shame, and stigma to increase understanding and provide the different types of care that different people need to achieve healthier outcomes mentally, emotionally, behaviorally, and physically—not just for one, but for all.

Various developmental and health conditions can impact the neurology and physiology of your brain and body, which impact how the amygdala and prefrontal cortex develop and operate. Whatever the developmental differences, the functional importance of these parts of the brain remain the same, even when certain functions may be more or less challenging for some than others.

Autism Spectrum Disorder (ASD) – Generally speaking, ASD is a developmental disorder of variable severity that is characterized by difficulties in social interaction and communication, and by restricted or repetitive patterns of thought and behavior. Symptoms of ASD can vary among individuals, from those with very few or less severe symptoms or difficulties, to those with multiple or more severe symptoms and difficulties.

Research also indicates that the neurological differences associated with Autism tend to affect males more than females, although the findings have yet to be fully understood or explained—whether due to chromosomal or hormonal differences, or due to certain behavioral traits being associated more with men than women, that may be due to social and environmental influences as well.

Fetal Alcohol Spectrum Disorders (FASDs) – Fetal Alcohol Spectrum Disorders are a range of developmental conditions caused when any amount of alcohol passes through the blood stream to a developing fetus during pregnancy. The type of developmental disorder depends on the timing of the exposure during fetal development, but one of the most common symptoms is impaired brain development, most notably the prefrontal cortex.

Someone with an FASD may or may not have any physical symptoms, so the only way to diagnose an FASD is through behavioral observation, in addition to confirming that alcohol was in fact consumed during pregnancy. That's really the only way to diagnose an FASD with certainty. Without confirmation of prenatal exposure to alcohol, it's impossible to diagnose an FASD, since no other blood or genetic testing is yet available. For reasons still unknown, FASDs also tend to affect those born male more than those born female.

It's important to note that fetal brain development can also be affected by exposure to other drugs, chemicals, and even elevated levels of certain neurochemicals (especially associated with chronic stress), that can only be diagnosed through similar observational and self-reporting methods.

Dementia – Why do I include dementia under the topic of neurodiversity? It may seem controversial to some to include a neurodegenerative disease of the brain when discussing brain health, function, and development, since dementia cannot be treated with traditional mental health therapies. That said, many people still live and thrive with dementia, long before they may even be diagnosed, so it's important to be aware of the neurological signs and symptoms, as much as the mental fitness practices used to prevent and manage the condition, with greater understanding of brain health and function.

For a number of reasons, the same stigma that surrounds mental and neurological conditions also surrounds dementia. This may be in part due to the mental, emotional, and behavioral nature of symptoms associated with personality traits that tend to define one's sense of self and identity.

It's critical to be aware of brain health and function in every person in every capacity to combat the fear, shame, and stigma, often perpetuated by our disjointed healthcare system.

While every part of your brain and body are interconnected and function together as a whole organism, our healthcare system still treats the body as separate independent parts— often separating mental function from brain function as well— with specialists assigned to each who often don't learn together, work together, or agree on healthcare practices and treatment.

Whether this is due to how we educate and insure, or how different specialty areas compete for funding, I'm not sure.

What I do know, is that the same mental fitness practices used to prevent and manage mental, emotional, behavioral, and physical health conditions are the same used to prevent and manage symptoms of Alzheimer's and dementia.

Is this ironic? Absolutely not, since they all involve the brain.

The contributing neurological and physiological factors remain the same, including the neurological and physiological effects of stress, emotions, repetition, reinforcement, sleep, diet, and exercise.

Thankfully, through repetition and emotional reinforcement (via neurochemicals), the effects of learning music, dance, and other routine behaviors become unconsciously tethered to our long-term memory in our autonomic nervous system—what we often call "muscle memory."

This is why you remember songs you sing and hear over and over again, repetitive movements, and even routine behaviors like walking, biking, or driving, that become nearly automatic with practice and no longer require much conscious effort.

Since the autonomic nervous system is also connected to the amygdala (that drives your unconscious stress response), stress can equally exacerbate neurological conditions that compromise the prefrontal cortex—whether due to imbalance, injury, illness, or impairment—which is why stress management is such a critical part of promoting brain health and function in everyone.

It's important to know that the symptoms of dementia are similar to other mental health conditions, neurological conditions, diseases, and disorders, since dementia impacts the very organ that drives your mental processes—the brain.

Why is it important to include dementia in discussions of neurodiversity and mental fitness?

Mental fitness practices that promote brain health can also help reduce the risk of brain disorders and diseases, which is why prevention is as important as healing, treatment, or management after a diagnosis.

When we have a better understanding of the neurology of brain function, we also have a better understanding of how to care for those diagnosed with neurodegenerative diseases like dementia, that often impact the prefrontal cortex first. Minimizing and managing the unconscious stress response of the amygdala is a critical part of caring for someone diagnosed with dementia. When functions of the prefrontal cortex are increasingly impaired or inhibited, the unconscious stress response becomes even more powerful (which is why access to short-term working memory becomes harder while long-term memories may remain longer).

Even the most mentally fit people can find caregiving extremely challenging, which is why jobs that demand such high levels of emotional stress must also ensure sufficient time and care to rest and recover, to optimize performance. Minimizing and managing the unconscious stress response of caregivers is critical for providing proper care, since caregivers experience unusually high levels of emotional stress when caring for someone who is easily agitated, triggered, and confused due to a disease, disorder, or imbalance.

By promoting brain health and neurodiversity, we can empower every individual to feel and do their best by fostering healthful and supportive education, relationships, and environments.

Post-Traumatic Stress Disorder (PTSD) – When you experience a severe emotional trauma, it can essentially burn a neurological scar into your long-term memory and autonomic nervous system that requires tremendous therapeutic effort to treat and heal. In the brain of someone with PTSD, an unconscious stress response can be more easily activated by thoughts or sensations that trigger traumatic memories, emotions, and experiences, impairing healthful brain function and regulation, including critical functions of the prefrontal cortex that can affect overall health, safety, and well-being.

Every brain processes and stores information slightly (or very) differently, which is why the emotional experiences, perceptions, and beliefs of one can differ so much from the emotional experiences, perceptions, and beliefs of another.

Much like physical health, mental and behavioral health have many underlying factors that require proper care and understanding, including brain health. This is what makes understanding brain health so vital as part of your overall health and well-being—because physical health is dependent on behavioral health, that is dependent on mental health, that is dependent on brain health and function.

It's imperative to understand and care for your brain as part of your body, rather than a separate independent part, that is often the result of our specialized healthcare system. For example, your dentist might tell you to floss more—that requires a change in your behavior to form a new healthful habit—but if you struggle with a mental health condition or neurological difference, changes to your routine and forming new behaviors might be harder for you, that your dentist is not licensed to identify.

Mental fitness promotes healthful attitudes and behaviors based on scientific discoveries of how the brain operates, including the differences between people, to better understand the ways we process and filter information neurologically and physiologically in the brain.

As humans, we share a lot of the same feelings, but how and when we feel them and what triggers them can be as different as our DNA. It's those differences that can complicate our relationships when we can't see into our own brain or the brains of others. When the only way we can express what we think and feel is through words and behaviors (that don't always come easily), it can be even harder when our unconscious stress response has control over how we think, feel, and behave.

The only life we really know is our own. Therefore, we cannot expect others to understand our life experience if we do not share it, nor can we understand or speak for the life experience of another without inquiry, listening, and being in a mental state to comprehend and empathize.

This is why any effort to embrace diversity and inclusion requires mindfulness, emotional awareness, creativity, curiosity, and critical thinking—to engage the prefrontal cortex in a way that helps calm the amygdala.

When the prefrontal cortex is impaired or not fully developed—whether or not the condition has been properly identified or diagnosed—functions of the prefrontal cortex may also be impaired or underdeveloped, leading to difficulty in comprehension, performance, emotional regulation, impulse control, empathy, creativity, and even relating socially to other people.

This impairment also makes stress responses stronger and harder to regulate, that can make even minor changes to one's environment or routine extremely stressful and difficult to manage. Sensations and emotions may be harder to regulate and understand as well, seeming irrational when the unconscious stress response is stronger than their conscious impulse control and emotional regulation.

When an individual feels that their feelings are irrational and cannot be trusted, they may feel they are a threat to themselves or others that can lead to a whole host of other mental health challenges, with painful thoughts, feelings, and emotions, in a highly imbalanced and toxic state.

It's important to know that pain is pain, and is a serious neurological signal, whether in the brain or the body. The sensation of a stress, threat, harm, illness, or injury may be experienced differently by different people, but whether we experience it physically or emotionally, it is a neurological signal just the same that must be taken seriously.

If you are struggling with any of these complex thoughts, feelings, or emotions, please speak with a licensed medical healthcare provider or therapist who can help you identify, manage, or heal your neurological condition and help you find and maintain a more healthful balance.

Like every other part of your body, your brain function may be more or less active depending on a number of internal influences, including general health, age, and genetics. Body function and neurological connections are also reinforced with repetitive use—much like blazing a trail in your nervous system

Similarly, when certain body functions or neurological connections are less developed, the brain and body often strengthen other neurological connections to achieve a more balanced state. This is a process known scientifically as *neuroplasticity*, when different neuropathways form as a workaround with repetitive use. This is why one's sense of hearing might become stronger with the loss of vision, as they depend more on their hearing, and strengthen those neurons with repetitive use.

Neuroplasticity certainly is not a cure-all, but it's another way your brain and body adapt to achieve homeostasis—or a more balanced state—to operate in the most efficient and effective way possible, even when faced with a tremendous challenge.

Even when you're not aware of it, you deal with unconscious stress and change every day. There may be changes to your environment, body chemistry, thoughts, feelings, family life, work responsibilities, relationships, etc. Some changes may be healthful in that they help you heal, grow, and develop, while others may be unhealthful by impairing your healing, growth, and development.

There will certainly be ups and downs since we are not static beings, and your body chemistry can fluctuate for so many reasons each and every day. Even when you cannot control the changes, you can still try to understand them, to learn how to maintain a more balanced and healthful state—neurologically and physiologically, hormonally and metabolically.

It's less about "embracing change" and more about "embracing challenge," in order to identify and understand healthful change from unhealthful change—like the difference between selling your home (stressful with a healthful benefit) or being evicted (stressful with no healthful benefit). Both involve a different kind of change with a different kind of stress that requires a different kind of preparation and response.

Fitness is about developing the abilities you need to navigate both the healthful and unhealthful changes and challenges in life, in a healthful way, by understanding what influences your thoughts, feelings, and behaviors—so you can better manage your stress response, to feel and do your best, to achieve your goals, even in the face of great adversity.

MENTAL INFLUENCES

5 S.E.N.C. INVENTORY

Your brain health and mental functions are continually influenced by a combination of internal and external factors—including social, environmental, nutritional, and chemical influences that affect those electrochemical signals that transmit throughout your brain and body (otherwise known as your neurology and physiology).

I use the acronym S.E.N.C. (with artistic license to pronounce it as "sense") as a way to make it easier to remember all of the different kinds of sensory information and influences that impact your human brain and body, inside and out.

Mental influences are most often unconscious emotional influences that affect how you think, feel, and behave. So well-being isn't so much a matter of "mind over matter" as "minding what matters," starting with emotional awareness, especially when it comes to navigating your unconscious stress response.

It's often less about what or who is influencing you as how whoever or whatever makes you feel, inside and out, that's actually an unconscious emotional response. Just as you can have an unconscious emotional or stress response to people, you can also have unconscious emotional or stress responses to what you see, what you smell, what you touch, what you taste, and what you hear, whether a color, song, fragrance, food, chemical, animal, technology, lighting effect, fabric, air or water temperature, or even the weather.

Due to how your unconscious emotional response works neurologically as part of your autonomic nervous system, you are more likely to remember how you felt (i.e. happy, sad, excited, confused, etc.) than the specifics of what was actually said or done as well, since your unconscious emotional response is directly connected to your long-term memory.

This is why it can be so hard to identify and resist unhealthy influences when they make you feel good in the short-term, especially when it comes to unhealthy foods, chemicals, and even relationships. You may not realize the unhealthy effects until long after the initial enjoyment, after the pleasurable experience has been embedded in your long-term unconscious memory, which makes it harder for your conscious mind to remember and resist, when your unconscious mind only remembers those heightened emotions. This is in part why certain things can become addictive, by the neurochemical nature of emotions.

Developing healthier habits can be harder due to this neurochemical response as well, since you may have an unpleasant experience with something healthy that might be more challenging and stressful, or more bitter than sweet, until you experience the health benefits or develop a taste for it, when it evokes a sense of pleasure that makes it more enjoyable and easier for you to choose or do.

Remembering lists, names, or details that do not evoke an emotional response are harder to remember over the long term, which is why we need to repeat them to "memorize" them by consciously firing those conscious short-term neurons over and over again to reinforce them. This is also why an effective strategy for memorizing lists and names is to use a song, imagery, or word association to consciously tap into your emotional long-term memory.

So why don't we talk more about emotional influence and all the ways it is used (and abused)?

When you realize that your emotions are your own to manage, you empower yourself to take better emotional care of yourself and others as well.

You may be familiar with the Golden Rule that advises treating others how you want to be treated, and you might realize now how that requires engaging your prefrontal cortex. Similarly, you might also be familiar with the newer iteration commonly called the Platinum Rule, which builds on the Golden Rule by treating others how they want to be treated, which first requires engaging your prefrontal cortex to listen, learn, and respect them just as you would want them to listen, learn, and respect you. Both of these practices are stress-reducing in both you and them, by fostering a sense of respect, trust, and safety.

The Rusty Rule, however, is the term I use to describe the common practice of treating others how you think they "deserve" to be treated, often by how they treated you or others (especially when they treat you or others in a way you or they do not want to be treated). The Rusty Rule is a toxic form of spite or vengeance, driven by our unconscious stress response, that triggers the unconscious stress response in others.

This is stress-induced way of treating others is related to the old "eye for an eye" theory of justice and punishment, in which one feels justified in treating another the way they were treated. This toxic practice is self-perpetuating, due to the way our brains work. We are more likely to remember the harm done to us than the harm we do to others, since our amygdala (and long-term memory) is triggered by painful emotion, and empathy is inhibited when our amygdala is triggered as well. We often feel a sense of victory (with a rush of dopamine) when we harm or otherwise inhibit that or those we perceive as a threat, which reinforces our feelings and behaviors..

Much like a magic trick, once you become consciously aware of the unconscious emotions involved, you are also less easily influenced by those attempting to manipulate your unconscious emotions and stress response to influence your thoughts, feelings, and behaviors. Once the illusion of emotional manipulation is shattered, so is their power of influence.

Whether the influencer is an advertiser, religious leader, or politician, or even a friend, colleague, or family member, those who want to maintain mental and emotional control over you do not want you to be conscious of your unconscious emotional response, and the unconscious emotional influence they have over you. This is also why those who are attempting to manipulate you do not like it when their influence is challenged by asking, "WHY?"

Asking why is a conscious effort to understand and comprehend, that reduces our unconscious stress response and powers up our prefrontal cortex that fuels empathy, emotional regulation, and impulse control.

What makes manipulative influences even harder to consciously spot, challenge, and identify is when the one attempting to emotionally manipulate you is also a source of emotional comfort for you, that is the source of their power.

This is why it can be particularly hard to be consciously aware of emotional manipulation when we feel a sense of safety, trust, connection, and affection for the one who is emotionally manipulating us.

The process of manipulatively building that emotional sense of safety, trust, connection, and affection for abusive purposes is what's known as "grooming."

The shattering of an emotional illusion can also be quite emotionally painful as your neurons are forced to fire differently, to adapt to the new perception of reality you have, and no longer stimulate the neurochemicals that at one time had elicited a soothing sense of emotional reward (namely dopamine). Your sense of trust, faith, hope, and safety can feel completely lost by the resulting unconscious stress response that is part of the grieving process, and why it can neurologically feel so painful—as painful as physical pain that is neurological just the same.

Do you have a favorite friend, family member, food, drink, sports team, band, brand, app, game, book, or movie?

If so, that is the result of mental and emotional influence— more specifically your unconscious neurochemical response. The influence isn't so much about how your favorite things consciously make you think, but how they unconsciously make you feel. That unconscious emotional response is what influences our likes, preferences, desires, and biases— neurologically and physiologically.

When we are challenged to accept that someone (or something) we like, trust, or even love is being emotional abusive or manipulative, our unconscious stress response can trigger a defensive state as a form of grief, with waves of denial, anger, anxiety, bargaining, anxiety, and depression.

Grief is never a linear process, and involves many complex emotions and even combinations of, due to your unconscious neurology and neurochemistry. The neurons in your unconscious mind are forced to change and reroute when they no longer evoke feelings of joy and comfort, but rather pain and distress. Grief is the neurological process that your brain goes through to adapt to a stressful or threatening state, that includes adjusting to the loss of a loved one, the loss of a home, the loss a job, the end of a marriage, or any other change that no longer evokes the same sense of trust, safety, comfort, and well-being that once was.

This unconscious neurochemical response is why we often first resist a challenging change or information that we perceive as threatening, whether as anger or denial, due to the emotional (neurological) pain or discomfort we feel. This is also why we tend to defend (and grieve) that and those we love more than that and those we don't—since we experience a greater neurochemical stress response when that or those we love are harmed, lost, or threatened.

Due to how our neurochemistry works, we consume what we like and reject what we don't—even when it might be good for us. While we are becoming wiser consumers of food—by asking what's in it, how it was prepared, and where it was produced—we are still junkies when it comes to the information we consume, that often fuels our unconscious stress response.

The problem is that it's often hard to tell the difference between healthful and unhealthful influences when the unhealthful things make us instantly feel good, even when it makes us feel crappy later. Our neurology doesn't associate that delayed response, whether delayed punishment or gratification. This makes it much harder to develop healthful habits when the gratification, gain, or reward is delayed.

The degree to which you like or desire something can ebb and flow as well, depending on your neurochemical response.

For example, imagine not seeing someone you love for a long time, and how you feel when you see them again—that rush of good feelings. Now imagine how you feel seeing that same person every day and night. Do you feel the same rush of good feelings? Likely not because your neurochemicals rebalance, and you acclimate to them being in your environment. That doesn't mean you don't still love them, but that rush of emotion after not seeing them is not the same as how you feel seeing them day after day, when your unconscious stress response may be triggered as well, either by something they said or did, or by something else that has nothing to do with them.

The same goes with other things that bring you pleasure in life too—like your favorite food, song, movie, or game. When we haven't experienced it in a while, we get a rush of feel-good neurochemicals like serotonin, dopamine, or oxytocin (to name a few major ones). After the fifth, twentieth, or hundredth time in a row eating it, listening to it, watching it, or playing it, however, we no longer feel that rush of good feelings and excitement once we acclimate, and may actually get tired or bored of it when it no longer stimulates that rush of good feeling it once did.

When we go without it for a while, and our neurochemicals acclimate again without it, we will likely feel that rush of pleasure again when we experience it again. This is why we often say, "Absence makes the heart grow fonder," and, "We don't know what we have until it's gone."

Your true power may go unnoticed too, until it's gone.

Ultimately, your power is not your ability to control, but rather your ability to influence behaviors, choices, decisions, and outcomes—including how you influence your own success, health, and well-being. What makes one truly powerless, is not their lack of control but their lack of influence, their inability to navigate a situation—even when it's not within their control—to get where they want to go.

When we fail to realize the power of influence, we can confuse power with control, of which we have very little in life. It's this lack of control that can make us feel powerless, when we don't realize the power in our ability to influence. Think of someone you consider powerful. Do they really have control that is 100 percent certain, or do they have the ability to influence outcomes, that comes with some risk and uncertainty?

On the flip side, when we believe in someone else's power and abilities more than our own, we give away our power (and responsibility) to them.

For example, when someone says or does something that triggers your unconscious stress response that spoils your mood and ruins your day, that is their power over you. However, when you develop the ability to manage your own unconscious stress and process your thoughts and feelings in a healthful way, to not let what someone else says or does spoil your mood and ruin your day, then their power is weakened and yours is increased.

You need and deserve healthful influences to be well and happy, that starts by caring for yourself. Every moment of every day is a new opportunity to be aware, to choose, to begin again. It's up to you to understand what influences you, and how to manage your unconscious stress response, to find the healthful influences you need.

Your time and attention are probably the most precious non-renewable resource on Earth—that is what's bought and sold every minute of every day, to employers, politicians, advertisers, and influencers—so be sure to spend your time and attention wisely, to promote your own health and well-being (rather than just lining someone else's pockets).

This is one of the most challenging parts of life—to find the right balance of stress, responsibility, power, and control that fuels a healthful level of pride, reward, and motivation without feeling discouraged, anxious, or depressed—when the stress becomes too much.

In order to truly feel empowered—to have a sense of control and influence over the outcome—we must first take responsibility, that can also cause stress. With responsibility comes the risk of failure, criticism, and even humiliation. The risk associated with responsibility can trigger an unconscious stress response of fear, panic, or worry, and even discourage us from taking responsibility—giving up our power to someone else. This transfer of power might make things easier for us in the short-run by soothing our unconscious stress response, but may make it harder and more stressful in the long-run when we have little power or influence. When we have limited responsibility, we also have limited power and influence that also limits our sense of pride, purpose, reward, and motivation.

This might apply to work situations and even relationships, including parental power, influence, and responsibility.

When you realize your power is your ability to influence, you can take great pride in your power and feel motivated to take responsibility, as well as the results of your influence—that often come later than sooner. So when you're wondering about the power you have, remember that you likely have much more than you think, long before you might see the results.

It's nearly impossible to maintain a healthy attitude and healthy behaviors without believing we deserve it first, or believing we can, or understanding the work that it takes. It's like trying to drive cross-country on one tank of gas. It takes more than that. It doesn't happen just because we wish it or demand it. It happens with understanding, learning, and experience; by working through thoughts and feelings with intention, motivation, and positive reinforcement, by believing in ourselves and our abilities, to feel and do our best, because we deserve it.

It happens when we overcome the stigma around mental health, that has made us believe we must struggle on our own in order to prove our strength, independence, and self-reliance.

It happens when we stop the perception that seeking help is somehow shameful or weak, when in fact it is a sign of strength.

It happens when we broaden our definition of fitness beyond the body, to include the mind, because only when we care for our mind can we truly thrive.

As challenging as it can be, it's important to remember how interdependent and influenced we all are by each other, by our environment, by what we consume sensationally, informationally, nutritionally, and chemically, and the inner workings of our human brain and body. We are part of the same ecosystem and environment now more than ever in this global age that is largely driven by our global economy (i.e., money, power, and influence).

There's a reason why social media influencers get paid for the revenue they can generate by influencing the thoughts, feelings, and behaviors of others.

Without even knowing it, you could be influencing someone on the other side of the world with what you say, do, or create—while someone you've never met can just as easily influence you, without even being aware.

Do some people find bliss in their ignorance? For sure, especially when they aren't aware of the loss or harm, that prevents a stress response.

Does ignorance cause harm? Definitely, since we tend to cause greater injury when we aren't aware and don't know better.

Is it a conspiracy? Likely not, since we often don't realize the harm we do until after it's done, and most healthy individuals don't consciously want to feel the guilt or pain associated with being responsible for deliberate harm.

If for some neurochemical reason, we find pleasure in harming others (i.e., if we believe the ones we harm pose a threat to us), then premeditation and conspiracy could definitely be a possibility. We might even attempt to consciously justify our unconscious stress response, in order to avoid the feelings of guilt or pain associated with our behavior.

This is why shame is so unhealthy and ineffective when it comes to healing and resolve—that requires the function of your prefrontal cortex. Shame triggers our unconscious stress response in the amygdala that impairs our prefrontal cortex from higher functioning, required to balance and heal the neurochemistry of our mind and emotions.

The various forms of dysfunction that impact our health and well-being don't exist in a vacuum. They feed off of each other as part of a system.

When you feel good about yourself and care about yourself, you're less likely to turn to something unhealthy to make you feel better, because you feel motivated to take care of yourself, and can even find reward in caring for others. On the flip side, when you don't care for yourself, then you're more likely to turn to something unhealthy, and will find it harder to care for others (and may even feel jealous or resentful when you do).

Depending on your life experience and what others have told you, you might have an easier or harder time believing that you are valuable and significant just for being human. With every breath you take and action you make, you need and deserve proper care and protection, as much as every other part of nature, and every other person on the planet.

Your intrinsic value is in being part of nature, and in your humanity, that cannot be taken away by anyone's opinion or belief.

Just by being human, you are an important and significant part of nature just like every other plant, animal, and element—all of which are a part of you too, in every cell and fiber of your being. That might sound cheesy, but it's true. As much as we must care for and protect the environment, so must we care for and protect ourselves and each other as a significant part of it—the part that we so easily forget when we fight each other over who is right and who is wrong (due to how the human brain works).

So why do we struggle with valuing ourselves and each other?

It's in part related to how we also value money and power, relative to what we can do with it, that is constantly fluctuating through the power of economics based on supply and demand—what is rare versus what is in abundance. We tend to place greater value on what's limited more than what's plentiful, or the preferred taste, style, or fashion of the time. We value what's "new" and current more than what's "old" and outdated, until what's "old" becomes rare and desirable again. The value might increase or decrease based on what we like versus what we don't by comparison.

And our value system doesn't just apply to things, but people too.

The operative word in our value system being comparison, which is also known as the "thief of joy" due to the stress response involved.

Is it any wonder why the "pursuit of happiness" can be so elusive and fleeting when we focus so much on comparison to define our sense of worth and success, based on money and popularity, income and status, driven by stress and competition?

In our highly competitive money-driven culture, this value system directly influences how we value ourselves and each other.

This is one of the powers of perception, and the difference between intrinsic and extrinsic value. That is, the value that someone or something has naturally in and of themselves or itself (that cannot be measured in dollars or popularity) versus the value we place on someone or something, based on how others value it or them, and what we get in return, that can change over time (like celebrity status, precious gems, youth, or sex appeal).

Our power comes from how much influence we have, whether in the form of money or popularity, which is why we envy those who have more power, influence, money, and popularity than we do, especially when our sense of value is relative based on comparison. Our innate sense of value, power, and influence is therefore diminished by comparison when we perceive that others have more (that in a nutshell is what drives the "popularity=money" machine otherwise known as social media).

But while we so often associate money with power, money itself does not have power. Money is only worth as much as we value it and what it can buy us—that is, the influence it has on others to give us what we want.

We say "heavy is the head that wears the crown" because what's often not considered with the glamour of power, fame, and fortune is the added stress, expectation, responsibility, accountability, and criticism that often go along with it—and the unhealthful results when these added stressors are not managed in a healthful way.

We often say "with great power comes great responsibility" when we should also say "with great responsibility comes great power." For example, the President of the United States does not have power until they take on the responsibilities of being President. Similarly, no leader has great power until they take on the responsibility of being a leader. It's the responsibility bestowed onto a leader that makes them a leader.

Why am I telling you all of this?

Empowered people are those who are aware of their power and influence, who can manage their stress response to think carefully and critically for themselves, to navigate and choose wisely, who feel motivated to take responsibility—who are therefore less susceptible to emotional manipulation, by being aware of how and why they feel the way they do.

Believing in your own abilities is a critical step in empowerment. Even before that, though, perceiving that something is possible is the very first step toward achievement, before you even realize what you can do. When you lack healthful influences like a healthy role model or someone to teach you what you can do—to help build your self-confidence, to believe in your abilities, to feel and do your best—achievement can be even harder.

An important part of your success and well-being is to feel empowered, and to know what your power is—that is your ability to influence and navigate—that does not require money, fame, or even popularity, but does require responsibility and emotional intelligence to understand how human emotions work, as a function of the brain.

When we only focus on extrinsic rewards like money, fame, and popularity, we quickly lose sight of our intrinsic value and power that influences our sense of self and purpose. We can then feel powerless and hopeless without the level of money, fame, and popularity that we believe makes us powerful. We can lose sight of the very real power and influence we already have that is more important than any amount of money or popularity—that is our sense of self, our pride, and our integrity, that cannot be bought or sold. Nor can it be shamed out of us by those who feel threatened by our power, believing that it diminishes the value of their own by comparison (another consequence of our extrinsic value system based on relativity).

When we experience more stress than we expect, however, we may develop a fear of success and responsibility—choosing to give up our power and influence in exchange for less stress (a sense of powerlessness that comes with stress of its own).

By extrinsic standards, we are taught that happiness is having what we want, that is also never enough, since we no longer want what we have once we get it, once the dopamine and serotonin fade. We are constantly driven to want what we don't have through the influences of marketing, media, and social pressure. Our sense of self is too often determined this way too, by comparison of what others have and we don't, that makes us want it. We want to be the winner (of which there are few), because being a loser is shameful (of which there are many). We seek more money and popularity to feel superior, to be the best, to be the winner—because that's what we've been taught and told, that's been reinforced by our drivers of fear and reward.

Of course in today's world, you do need enough money and social support to provide basic needs and life essentials. We work our butts off to prove our worth, for validation and acceptance, for reward—to feel like our life has value, meaning, and purpose—because we fear the alternative of living a life with no value, no meaning, and no purpose, as determined by our highly competitive money-driven culture. Yet as hard as we work, we rarely feel that we have enough—and sadly, we often compare ourselves to those with less than we do, who legitimately do not have enough, in order to feel like we have enough.

When we realize the vicious cycle we're on, and feel we're never achieving that sense of happiness that we want (that is inhibited by stress), we can lose hope and motivation.

Fear and reward are the primary (and primal) forces that fuel every moment of every day as neurochemical functions of the brain.

Your ability to feel your best, to do your best, is essentially driven by these forces, that starts by shedding fear and shame to value and empower yourself, no matter your wealth or popularity.

There's just so much that influences your brain, your thoughts and feelings, your perception of reality, most of which are not conscious choices. You might even struggle with how you perceive yourself, that sense of knowing and loving who you are at your core, beyond what others think you are.

So let's take a step back and look under the hood at what drives it all.

Those crappy sensations you feel are signals telling your brain that some part of your system is out of balance and in need of care, whether at the structural level (like a muscle or joint issue) or at the cellular level (like a virus or chemical imbalance). Whatever is throwing off your system to make you feel that way, you first need to tune into how you feel, to figure out what it is that's causing that feeling, in order to heal, regain balance, and recover—that's not always easy, and often requires a healthcare specialist to help you figure it out.

Biologically, your brain processes information and experiences much like your stomach processes food—physiologically and neurologically—and just as digestive health is a functional aspect of gut health, so is mental health a functional aspect of brain health.

This is why it's so important to accept and understand the basics of how your brain and body work together to understand those signals and find the care and support you need.

Approaching mental health as a function of your brain can also help squash the toxic shame, stigma, and moral judgment that too often get in the way of finding proper care. Understanding the basics of your neurology and physiology empowers you to take better care of yourself by understanding what influences your thoughts, feelings, and behaviors in a non-judgmental way, to promote better health, healing, and well-being.

So it's time to flip fitness on its head.

Our modern healthcare system has divided up the body into so many separate parts, with a different healthcare provider specializing in one area or another. There are those who believe in one method of healthcare and not another. It's no wonder why taking care of ourselves can feel so complicated and confusing, when the very people who are trained and paid to help us don't even agree or know what's going on.

Just as your brain sends signals to your body consciously and unconsciously, there are a number of neurological signals from various areas of your body that impact your brain unconsciously as well, that require your conscious awareness to interpret and understand them, to make wise and healthful choices.

For example, your brain and gut are highly interconnected neurologically and physiologically, that's often referred to as your gut-brain connection. This is often why we even have a "gut sense".

When you understand the basic function and building blocks of your brain and body, you can take better care of yourself by understanding why you feel the way you do and the steps you need to take to feel and do your best.

When we have a choice between instant or delayed gratification, instant gratification is just too hard to refuse. The sweet spot is really when both methods are used together, when one enhances the other by both providing instant reward as well as long-term benefit.

This is really the basic goal of mental fitness—to promote healthful behaviors by increasing emotional awareness. From there, you can use that awareness to promote behaviors that will help you achieve your goals.

Do you have a goal in mind?

Having a specific, measurable, achievable, relevant, and timely goal (i.e., a S.M.A.R.T. goal) is a great place to start, since having a specific goal can help fuel your motivation neurochemically—with those feel-good neurochemicals like serotonin and dopamine. You might have a major life goal in mind, or your goal might be more modest and general, like just wanting to feel better. However big or small your goals are, it's important to think about the direction you want to go so you can prepare your brain and body for the work involved, to take those first important steps to get there—even if the first step is just getting out of bed.

Living healthfully is a goal in itself that restarts again each day, and also involves learning along the way.

6 STRESS AND MOTIVATION

Do you know what motivates you and why? What gives you that drive or sense of purpose? Are you driven by hope and healing, or fear and stress?

Depending on the situation, what drives your motivation may change, whether fueled by a hopeful dose of serotonin and dopamine or a stress-induced dose of cortisol and adrenaline. It's not a matter of right or wrong, but rather an understanding of the effect that it has on your health and well-being.

For example, in which situation would you run the fastest?

1) A hungry lion is chasing you.
2) A cheerleader is chasing you.
3) Nobody is chasing you.

Even when the ultimate goal in each situation is to maintain your health and well-being, your fear of being attacked and even eaten by a lion gives you the most immediate rush of adrenaline that fuels a surge of neurochemical energy through your autonomic nervous system. That is quite literally the path of least resistance, which is why it happens so fast. Your unconscious stress response requires no conscious effort and therefore requires no proactive effort or conscious energy that could delay your response, and put you at greater risk of being caught by the lion.

While reactively running for your life is good, proactively running for your health and well-being is even better—because it proactively prepares you for when you have to reactively run for your life too!

Finding motivation to run for your health and well-being requires conscious effort that is much harder to do and maintain. It takes more neurochemical energy to operate the conscious part of your brain, especially when you may be perfectly comfortable, relaxed, and stress-free on your couch (that requires no conscious effort either).

You are absolutely right to think that marketers, advertisers, and media developers know how powerful your unconscious stress response is too. There seems to be more and more pressure these days to remain scared and angry in an attempt to keep us engaged and motivated, rather than comfortable and complacent.

Encouragement and social support can really help increase motivation and performance as well, by stimulating a boost of serotonin and dopamine that increases your energy and motivation to maintain your health and well-being, by proactively engaging your prefrontal cortex. This is when a cheerleader, trainer, coach, or supportive friend, for that matter, can really help!

Uplifting music can also have a similar effect with how your brain and body respond to the tonality and rhythm of music, that give your brain a boost of neurochemicals, that increase your heart rate and energize you to move.

While an adrenaline rush from our unconscious stress response might be much easier to produce (and more addictive and intoxicating too), it also comes from stress and fear that can contribute to other unhealthful thoughts and feelings. Since stress also contributes to an increased level of cortisol in your system, it also contributes to an unbalanced neurological and physiological state that puts a lot of wear and tear on your cells and internal systems.

The difference between having a valid reason that must be understood versus using an excuse to avoid effort and accountability can also complicate the situation.

How often do we say that we don't want an "excuse" for "bad" (or unhealthy) behavior?

So let's unwrap this. Let's first consider the difference between a "reason" and an "excuse."

Probably the most infamous excuse is, "The dog ate my homework!"

If this is in fact a lie to get out of doing your homework, then it's obviously an excuse.

On the other hand, if your dog did, in fact, eat your homework because you left it on the floor where the dog could easily eat it (especially if it's happened before), is that a valid reason, or just an excuse?

In my professional opinion (self-proclaimed as the one writing this book), it might still seem like an excuse since there is accountability to be taken for leaving your homework on the floor, when you could've taken preventive measures to not have your homework get eaten. You still need to take accountability for not taking good care of your homework (especially if it's happened before).

However, if your dog legitimately ate your homework even after you took preventive measures by putting it safely on your desk in a folder, then that might qualify as a reason more than just an excuse, since you did take proper precautions and did not know the dog would be able to jump up and eat your paper (especially if it's the first time—the sneaky bugger).

One might argue that the dog's behavior is still your responsibility, since it's your dog, that might still classify it as an excuse. That said, if you learn from the experience and take proper precautions to make sure it doesn't happen again, then that would be the result of having a legitimate reason, for which you took accountability.

This goes for brain health and function as well. Sometimes there are reasons beyond our awareness, understanding, and control that result in unhealthful or undesirable outcomes. The best we can do is take accountability, by understanding the reason to take proactive preventive measures, to achieve more healthful outcomes. When we simply dismiss a reason as an excuse, then we miss the opportunity to learn and understand to achieve healthful outcomes.

Other times we might lie or formulate an excuse to not have to take accountability for our poor judgment or mistakes. We might even believe the excuse ourselves, since it comes so naturally as an unconscious stress response. It does not feel good in our human brain to admit wrongdoing or making mistakes, that could leave us vulnerable to criticism or attack (triggering our unconscious stress response).

Even when we don't like challenges in life, that does not mean those challenges are just excuses, but rather reasons we need to understand.

When we want people to tell us the truth, we need to foster a sense of trust and safety, so they can tell us the truth without fear of punishment, attack, or criticism (as long as learning the truth doesn't trigger our own unconscious stress response that validates their stress response as a reason to lie—talk about challenging!).

So why is brain health and mental function so much more difficult to accept and understand than physical health and body function?

When someone doesn't feel physically well and isn't able to perform their duties to the best of their abilities, we would likely advise they stay home to rest and recover, to see a doctor and take care of themselves.

When the very same person doesn't feel emotionally or mentally well enough to perform their duties to the best of their abilities, there's a high probability we would expect them to "shake it off," "let it go," or "get over it," and stop making excuses.

If someone isn't behaving in a healthful way, isn't it better to understand why, to help them understand their behaviors, to seek the care they need, to feel and do their best?

Isn't it better to help them learn and accept whatever challenges they face, rather than shaming them for the way their brain works?

Why do we so quickly jump shame and blame rather than acceptance and understanding when it comes to discussing thoughts and feelings?

In one word—STRESS.

Unfortunately, we as humans are driven by stress in many ways—it is often our primary means of increasing energy and motivation—by releasing cortisol and adrenaline that prepare your body for intense work. It's the demands and expectations we place on ourselves and each other that help keep many of the wheels in our society and economy in motion, and even add excitement through competition! Before we celebrate too hard, though, there's also a down-side to all of those demands, expectations, and competition too—as so often there's a yin to the yang.

We all want to feel accepted, valued, and appreciated—to feel safe and in charge of our own destiny. When we don't, we may feel threatened, triggering our amygdala and unconscious stress response.

There's a reason we have a stress response—to help us thrive and survive. With every goal there is an element of change, with every change there is an element of challenge, and with every challenge there is an element of stress.

A common motivator is finding a sense of purpose in life that is often fueled by stress—to solve a problem, achieve a goal, or meet a demand. It's a basic part of our survival instinct to be aware of, and reduce those dangers and threats to our safety and existence—to protect ourselves, our families, and our communities.

When we see each other as a threat, our stress response is triggered just the same, that can lead to separation, segregation, containment, incarceration, tribalism, aggression, violence, war, and even death—as a way to protect and defend against the threat.

When we see ourselves as a threat, or that the pain we feel is in itself a threat to our well-being, then our stress response can be directed at ourselves.

Have you noticed that even when life is going great, we still look for problems?

Due to our unconscious stress response, we tend to focus more on the problem than the resolve.

This is why relying on an adrenaline rush or other neurochemical booster or blocker to motivate us might trigger good feelings at the start, but can have long-term health consequences in the end.

Before there can be healthful, meaningful, and lasting change, there must be understanding of how to achieve and sustain it. It's not enough to point out the problem. It's like pointing at a car that doesn't work. It's not enough to kick it and curse at it. It's not even enough to open the hood unless we understand what's inside and how it operates. We must not only acknowledge but understand the problem before we can fix it.

Our greatest power really is our ability to influence, teach, inspire, motivate, and otherwise influence desired outcomes.

When we allow ourselves the time and space to be curious about the human brain (rather than judgmental or morally superior), we can reduce the fear, shame, and stigma that so often get in the way by triggering an unconscious stress response that impair the very functions of the brain we are trying to optimize. When we reduce stress, we can actually energize the higher-functioning conscious part of the brain to feel and do our best, as the uniquely complex organisms we are.

The healthier path to motivation requires conscious effort and practice, by promoting hope and healing to reduce stress and cortisol in your system, to achieve a healthier neurochemical balance. By being aware of how different influences affect your emotionally, and how to calm your amygdala to engage your prefrontal cortex, you can make healthier choices to improve and maintain your health and well-being.

When you're being chased by a wild animal, it's probably best to let your amygdala do its "fight or flight" thing!

But when you're fighting with a family member, friend, or colleague, or you have a tendency to freeze in fear, it's then wiser to calm your amygdala to engage your prefrontal cortex.

When fighting a problem becomes our sense of purpose, we can actually feel guilty for NOT feeling stressed—like we're not paying enough attention or trying hard enough—when in reality, solving the problem would actually mean reducing or eliminating the stress that stems from it.

Are you driven by stress? Are you fueled by hope or despair? Do you trust yourself and others? Do you embrace or fear success?

The challenge is that when we are driven by our stress response and the resulting adrenaline rush, our sense of purpose and motivation can fade along with the problem when it's finally resolved, creating a codependent relationship with problems that fuel our sense of purpose and motivation. This toxic cycle can be incredibly challenging to break, when we lose our conscious sense of hope and motivation to proactively maintain a healthful state, rather than being unconsciously motivated by the adrenaline rush that comes with reacting to a crisis in need of recovery.

As Americans, we tend to attribute being less stressed with not working hard enough, and assume that having an easy life lacks value and meaning.

We find purpose in our problems and are rewarded for it— that sustains our unhealthy addiction to stress, neurologically and physiologically speaking. We take great pride in our ability to overcome stressful challenges and obstacles, and often equate stress with how hard we work. We're told that we must work hard (with high levels of stress) to get results, recognition, and reward. We've been sold on the notion that the more stressed you are, the more important you are, and the more money you will make.

We sure do love to chase that carrot!

As Americans, we especially seem to have a complex relationship with stress, success, and the ability to maintain a healthful state. You may have been taught and told that you must work hard for the good life, that winning is everything, and that taking pride in your accomplishments is shameful, since we also tend to envy those who have more than we do by comparison (that is compounded by social media). Many of us develop a sense of shame and guilt when we achieve something since we were never taught that it's OK (and essential!) to relax and enjoy it.

We get paid to take on more stress, and therefore feel forced to choose between paying more to help manage our stress (i.e., hiring an assistant, babysitter, personal trainer, therapist, etc.) or working less in order to reduce stress, that may result in reduced pay and put our financial well-being at risk.

This unfortunate disparity between what drives our health (low stress) and what drives our economy (high stress) contributes to the health and economic inequities we face. When earning more money requires taking on more stress, and maintaining your health requires reducing stress, we're forced to choose between health and wealth. We are implicitly taught that we can have one or the other, but not both. When in reality, we need both—we need our health to maintain our wealth, and we need our wealth to maintain our health.

As previously mentioned, being motivated by fear and stress may be beneficial in the short-term, but can be toxic and unhealthy in the long-term. Chronic or prolonged heightened levels of cortisol in your system can have harmful effects on your brain and body (not to mention your relationships and environment), preventing you from regulating your emotions and body chemistry, or otherwise recovering from the neurological and physiological imbalance that stress produces.

Again, the reason fear and anger can be so effective at motivating people is because they trigger our unconscious stress response that requires no conscious effort.

This is also why fear and anger can be incredibly unhealthful and antisocial motivators as well, because of the chain reaction that goes along with it—including unconscious biases as well as inhibited empathy, critical thinking, emotional regulation, impulse control, and comprehension (that are powered by the prefrontal cortex).

Anger might motivate some to fight as a stress response driven by the amygdala, but anger does not lead to comprehension, critical thinking, or problem solving, that is driven by the prefrontal cortex. It's the power of trust and curiosity that helps calm the amygdala to engage the prefrontal cortex.

When your unconscious stress response is triggered, it's more difficult to think critically because the energy is being sucked away from your prefrontal cortex to power your stress response. We tend to shame people as a reaction to our unconscious stress response in an attempt to control whatever or whoever is posing a threat or stressing us out, expecting them to flee or freeze under the pressure of our threatening response, that triggers their unconscious stress response. Quite often, however, they fight back.

We so often jump to the conclusion that maintaining our health and fitness is just about controlling what and how we eat and exercise, and telling others how to eat and exercise, without understanding the underlying factors of behaviors. We tend to emphasize the importance of healthy habits without discussing the underlying mental and physical health factors that influence our neurology and physiology, including our metabolism.

We might struggle with obesity, an eating disorder, anxiety, depression, grief, loneliness, arthritis, metabolic or hormonal imbalances, or any combination of neurological or physiological factors that influence the way our body physiologically stores and uses energy, including elevated levels of cortisol that alter digestion and metabolism.

Add to it the social shame and stigma that compounds the stress and cortisol in our system, that impacts our mental, emotional, and metabolic state. It's a bit like trying to walk up an escalator that keeps pushing you down.

The belief that our thoughts, feelings, and behaviors are all in our conscious control, regardless of our neurological and physiological health and development, is one of the major contributing factors to the stigma that surrounds mental, emotional, and behavioral health.

This is why the stress-induced judgment of shame can be so harmful to your health.

The toxic shame and stigma that surrounds mental, emotional, and behavioral health teaches us to hide any thoughts, feelings, and emotions that may be judged as socially unacceptable or undesirable, that might make us seem weak or vulnerable.

As a result, we often turn to unhealthy means of venting, self-soothing, self-medicating, or even self-harm—whether through food, drugs, sex, anger, aggression, or other risky behaviors—in an attempt to reduce pain by increasing those pain-reducing neurochemicals like adrenaline, serotonin, and dopamine in less-than-healthful ways.

Since the prefrontal cortex is not fully developed until around the age of twenty-five, and may be otherwise impaired or underdeveloped, neither are the functions of the prefrontal cortex fully functional.

While Western culture tends to consider anyone over the age of 18 (or who looks it) a "young adult," neurologically speaking they are not yet adults. A young adult would more accurately be anyone just over the age of twenty-five, whose brain is fully developed, with the full power and functionality of their prefrontal cortex, that drives what we consider "mature" behavior. It would also be more accurate to describe humans between the ages of 18-25 as "old children," since their underdeveloped brains may find it difficult to operate in a "mature" way.

As a society, however, we tend to believe what we see, and since young post-pubescent humans can have the same size, shape, and sound as adults, we tend to perceive them as adults, and expect them to act like adults. This is also why we tend to struggle and feel triggered or disappointed, when they don't behave in a fully mature way.

When we don't acknowledge or understand the development and function of the human brain (even when we can't see it), we can do a lot more harm than good by placing unrealistic expectations on underdeveloped brains—since ignorance leads to error.

As a society, we tend to justify these emotional and behavioral expectations on ripening adolescents, once they can reproduce or cause serious physical and emotional harm, when they don't practice impulse control and emotional regulation that is powered by their underdeveloped prefrontal cortex. While practicing emotional regulation and impulse control with realistic and achievable goals can be healthful, setting unrealistic and unachievable goals is not.

So what is "bad" behavior? Do we mean unhealthy, immature, irresponsible, disruptive, or destructive?

Out of an abundance of good intention, we create rules to define and enforce "good" behaviors, reinforced by reward or discouraged by punishment, without understanding the neurological or physiological origins of behavior, or how they are driven in the brain.

What are we actually rewarding? And what are we actually punishing?

What we deem "bad" behaviors are often signs of an underlying issue, whether an underdeveloped brain, mental health condition, physiological imbalance, neurological disorder, or cognitive impairment. Other times, what we deem "bad" might be a very healthful, mature, and responsible behavior for that individual, that simply makes us feel "bad" because of our own unconscious stress response when they defy, challenge, or contradict our expectations, desires, or demands.

Deciding what's "good" or "bad" based on how it makes us feel personally is not the best way to determine healthful from unhealthful, especially when we ignore brain health and function that is really the driver of behavior.

For example, if you witnessed someone screaming, punching a wall, or shouting profanities, you may judge that behavior as bad, unhealthy, destructive, or otherwise immature—until you learn that they just received a terminal diagnosis, or were just told that a loved one died in a tragic accident.

This illustrates how our perception is limited by the information we have. When we ask why, and receive more information, we can perceive the emotional cause and behavioral effect. We can reduce our stress response by comprehending and empathizing with the person, by imagining how receiving traumatic news would trigger a stress response in us as well. We also don't take personal offense (as an unconscious stress response) when we understand that another's stress response is not directed at us, but is a result of the emotional pain they feel.

Conversely, if they were to scream directly at you, punch you, or shout profanities at you, your stress response would likely be triggered, and you would have a harder time feeling empathetic and understanding—though you might still try to manage your stress response by understanding the circumstances.

This is why mental fitness is all about the WHY.

Traumatic experiences are not limited to death and disease, nor are they limited to only those that we can personally understand and comprehend. Often another person's pain is very hard to understand and comprehend, in which case we might feel irritated (as part of our unconscious stress response) and may belittle or reject their feelings as being too sensitive, childish, or immature (adding insult to injury in the process).

Emotional trauma does not leave our neurological system within an hour or two either, or even within a day, month, or year—and may even last a lifetime. We might even experience the unconscious effects of childhood trauma as adults. Traumatic experiences remain with us neurologically because of how the brain works, unconsciously connected to our autonomic nervous system and long-term memory.

This is why understanding brain health as the driver of behavioral health, emotional health, and mental health is so important to seeking, finding, and providing proper care, healing, and health management, including preventive care practices that proactively support healthy brain function, that is the focus of mental fitness.

In my years of research and business development, I have rarely heard mental health professionals discuss basic brain health and function. Similarly, in my dealings with brain health specialists, I have actually learned of efforts to disassociate brain health from mental health, in an attempt to reduce the stigma around neurological diseases that surrounds mental illnesses—rather than trying to reduce the stigma of brain health and function altogether.

It very much seems that while mental health professionals want nothing to do with brain health, brain health professionals also want nothing to do with mental health.

Does that make sense to you?

It sure doesn't make sense to me, and makes me ask the all-important question of WHY?

We're being told to develop healthy habits, eat healthy, and exercise—even when we have limited time, motivation, access, and resources—and while our own medical community doesn't agree on how the brain drives behaviors neurologically and physiologically. So we're told, "JUST DO IT!"

It's funny (as in not funny) how pretty much every mental health condition, neurological disorder, and cognitive impairment share many of the same symptoms often classified as "bad" behaviors— from attention deficit to hyperactivity, from emotional outbursts to inappropriate behavior, from eating disorders to sexual addiction, from drug abuse to physical aggression, from self-harm to suicide—all due to imbalanced or impaired brain function that relates to brain health and development, not an unhealthy spirit.

Simply put, we cannot achieve healthful outcomes when we

ignore basic brain health and development, and disassociate mental health and function from brain health and function— the very driver of behaviors, comprehension, impulse control, emotional (neurochemical) regulation, and stress management. When we are quick to shame (as an unconscious stress response) and slow to understand (that requires activation of the prefrontal cortex), we create a toxic self-perpetuating cycle of human dysfunction.

When a healthful choice or behavior triggers your unconscious stress response because you find it too difficult or challenging, you likely won't do it unless you have a conscious reason to energize your prefrontal cortex to make the conscious effort (often referred to as "willpower" or "motivation," depending on the circumstance).

This has nothing to do with being a "bad" or "weak" person; it's just how the human brain works, and why it's important to ensure proper care, training, and development.

That's not to say that stress is "good" or "bad" either, or that everyone experiences stress in the same way, since we are all diverse complex beings living diverse complex lives. This is, in part, the importance of understanding neurodiversity, to understand yourself and others from the inside out as fellow human beings.

Rather than placing value judgments on people, behaviors, or characteristics as "good" or "bad," we'll instead differentiate between "healthful" and "unhealthful," especially when it comes to healthful and unhealthful influences.

Stress is a natural part of life and cannot be avoided. There are all sorts of stressors in life, and struggling with stress is nothing to fear or be ashamed of, because it is just part of being human. Some stress can even be healthful when it creates a sense of excitement and motivation that leads to healthful outcomes. It's how you navigate stress that often differentiates healthful from unhealthful outcomes.

The main problem with stress is when it overwhelms your system and puts unhealthy wear and tear on your neurology and physiology, including your cells and organs, especially when stress is constant and chronic, sustained over long periods of time.

When you have an unhealthy dependence on stress as a motivator, it can create a toxic cycle of unhealthy influence that can be hard to change without conscious effort and practice. When fear and stress is what motivates you, you can actually develop an unconscious stress response to the very experience of success and achievement. This can prevent you from feeling that healthful sense of joy and accomplishment in your success (driven by a healthful release of serotonin and dopamine, that requires activation of your prefrontal cortex to comprehend and appreciate your achievement).

Depending on your upbringing and social environment, you might feel scared, guilty, or even unworthy of achievement, especially if those around you are quick to shame, judge, or otherwise express jealousy of your accomplishment (due to their own unconscious competitive stress response). Their unconscious stress response thereby reinforces your unconscious stress response.

In order to overcome this sense of stress from success, you may rely on feelings of anger and aggression, as part of your stress response, to stay motivated with that rush of cortisol and adrenaline.

Relying on stress as a motivator can also backfire when it leads to a fear of failure. When your fear of failure becomes so overwhelming that you inhibit the powers of your prefrontal cortex, you can actually unconsciously sabotage yourself as a way to reduce the stress that comes from failure by expecting failure. This unconscious stress response might manifest in thoughts that you are not good enough or worthy enough to win or succeed, and that even if you win, people will still criticize, reject, or attack you, which further impairs your motivation, confidence, and desire to succeed, or even try—when you fear both failure and success.

It's no wonder why it can feel like your head is spinning when you don't know how to get "unstuck" from this toxic mental cycle.

What differentiates you as a human from other animals, however, is your ability to understand yourself, and to be aware of your own emotions by using the powers of your prefrontal cortex—that must be continually nourished, nurtured, and exercised to fully function and develop.

When you feel stressed, your powers of empathy, comprehension, critical thinking, emotional regulation, and impulse control are all compromised as well, since energy essentially gets sucked up by your amygdala before it energizes your prefrontal cortex. Your brain gets backed up by stress in a way similar to how stress backs up your gut function as well, since it's all connected.

Your brain and body need healthful ways to release the toxic effects of stress that build up in your system. By activating your prefrontal cortex with mental fitness practices, you can lower the unconscious stress response of your sympathetic nervous system to activate the "rest, digest, rebalance, and repair" functions of your parasympathetic nervous system that unconsciously runs throughout your brain and body as well.

The key isn't to avoid your fears, but to be aware of them and address them, to find a healthful way to navigate through them—whether a fear of death, fear of failure, fear of success, fear of criticism, fear of rejection, fear of responsibility, or any other combination of fears that come along with being human that inhibit you from feeling and doing your best.

One way to reduce stress is with humor. By not taking this often confusing and irrational experience of being human too seriously, you can naturally reduce your stress response too (while being mindful to not trigger the stress response in others, as humor can be perceived in different ways). Genuine laughter that is not at the expense of another's feelings is a great stress reducer because it releases a healthful bit of endorphins, dopamine, oxytocin, and even serotonin into your nervous system, that all help calm your amygdala to energize your prefrontal cortex.

Fostering an environment in which you feel free to laugh and be your true authentic self is an important way to reduce social and environmental stress, that must include allowing others who share the environment to do the same, to reduce their stress response as well.

7 POWER OF PERCEPTION

How often have limiting thoughts or feelings gotten in the way of you feeling and doing your best (or even making an attempt)?

You may have been told that you can achieve anything you set your mind to if you just believe in yourself, but it sure helps when others believe in you too. When it comes to feeling and doing your best, it's rarely your potential or physical abilities that hold you back, but those limiting thoughts and feelings that influence your perception and the actions you take (or don't).

Your social environment directly influences your mental well-being, including how you think, feel, and behave, and how you perceive yourself, your abilities, and the possibilities around you.

Diversity, equity, inclusion (D.E.I.), and well-being are interconnected in their aim to influence healthful attitudes and behaviors—to empower every individual to feel and do their best, including YOU. Yet workplace wellness and D.E.I. programs are often separate, underutilized, and ineffective with another commonality—a general lack of awareness or understanding of how attitudes and behaviors form and function in the brain, neurologically.

This fact didn't really dawn on me until I first volunteered with a creative mentor program for inner-city kids called Art Buddies. What had originated as a program to expose kids to the power of creativity and creative careers, was really an unintentional form of art therapy that tapped into the power of perception.

At that point in my career, I had also been considering leaving my corporate communications job to start my own design business. I was ready for a leadership role that did not exist in the highly regimented and limited corporate structure.

What held me back, however, wasn't my lack of passion or abilities, but my self-doubt and fear of failure. I wasn't sure I could do it, or if I would regret leaving my comfortable corporate job to take that risk. My parents were self-employed as well, but as a kid, all I knew was the stress and uncertainty of self-employment, with constant worries about money, without the stability of a steady paycheck or affordable health insurance.

While volunteering with Art Buddies, I met all kinds of self-employed creative professionals who were making it on their own as entrepreneurs, including freelance designers, writers, photographers, and marketing professionals.

I knew that I needed a healthful change and challenge to keep growing and developing my life in the way I wanted, not just the way the company that I worked for wanted. Seeing others my age succeeding in a way that I wanted really changed my perception of what was possible, and what I could do too.

By meeting people much like me, with similar backgrounds and experiences, who had taken the leap and succeeded, I started to believe more in myself, including what I could do and what was actually possible. After a few years of considering the idea, I finally took the leap and left my comfortable corporate job of over ten years to start my own multimedia communications and design firm (yikes!).

Ironically, this was exactly the influence that Art Buddies mentors had on the children they worked with as well. By exploring their own creativity with adults who used creative skills in their work, the kids were able to believe in the value of their creativity by seeing how adults used creativity like theirs in different jobs too, that opened their minds to a range of career possibilities they had never considered before.

A few years after starting my freelance design firm and helping expand the Art Buddies mentor program, I jumped at the opportunity to become their next Executive Director. This opportunity would not have been possible had I remained in my old corporate job. It took three months for the Art Buddies board to make their final decision, and another six months of part-time training under the founder until I officially took over full-time—that was only made possible by the power and influence I had in running my own freelance business.

The next revelation in my "power of perception" discovery came when tasked with recruiting hundreds of adults to be creative mentors each year. I was amazed by how often adults would say, "I can't do that. I'm just not creative."

Time and again I found myself trying to convince adults (not kids!) that they were creative enough to be an Art Buddy!

That really got me wondering why that was.

Why do we become more self-conscious and less confident in our abilities after puberty? Why do we become afraid of failure, rejection, and defeat? Do we limit our perception of what we can do or become with grades, competitions, and awards granted only to the top few by comparison?

Are we too quick to focus on what we excel at and receive praise and reward, and less on what needs more practice and development through trial and error? Do we stop challenging ourselves for the sake of self-preservation and social acceptance as we age and define ourselves in limiting ways? Do we beat out that sense of wonderment, imagination, and fearlessness with a sense of shame, rejection, and belittlement when we fail, lose, or make a mistake?

To achieve any goal, you must first perceive the possibility to believe you can, to do what it takes to get there. The power of perception is in the influence of mentors, role models, and representation—as well as branding, marketing, media, and advertising—that influences our perception of who we are, what we can do, and what we can become. I refer to this process of discovery as "perceive, believe, achieve."

Perception influences your sense of reality, because your sensations are experienced by you alone, just as reality is perceived by every other individual in their own way, through their own senses and mental processes.

Your perception of reality also influences your identity and sense of self (i.e., your self-perception) that influences your values and sense of purpose in life, that can also create conflict between individuals with different life experiences and perceptions.

Similarly, when trying to reach diverse people with diverse backgrounds, education, and experiences (not to mention diverse genetics and neurology), there is never one language, one belief system, or one fitness practice that fits all. The same words, concepts, and practices can result in different neurological responses in the brains of different people, and may be interpreted and perceived differently depending on their knowledge or past experience.

You might even experience a sense of stress and unease when someone speaks a different language or uses words that you don't understand, especially when you don't know or trust the person and have nobody to explain or translate for you. Your brain hears the sounds but cannot make sense of them, that can cause an unconscious stress response when you can't understand it and perceive the lack of information as a threat to your sense of safety and security.

You might feel anxious, nervous, or afraid in that moment, and might pay more attention to their body language and physical cues to decipher their meaning. The unconscious stress you feel can also unconsciously impact your muscles and body movements, including your facial expressions and behaviors.

Your conscious mind might react by wondering (or saying aloud, if your impulse control and emotional regulation is inhibited by stress), "What are they saying? Is it something important? Are they talking about me? Should I be concerned? How can I communicate with them to ensure my safety?"

Conflict is essentially neurological friction caused by experienced differences. Just as physical friction occurs when two surfaces rub against each other in opposite directions, a similar neurological result happens when two people with opposing perceptions or perspectives interact. When we have a conflict with someone, we often say "they rub us the wrong way." When the reality that one perceives is different from the reality perceived by another, it can cause neurological friction.

Is reality always binary? Is one always right and the other always wrong? Or is reality someplace in the middle? Maybe reality is a combination of facts, viewpoints, and perspectives like viewing a globe, requiring input from all sides to get the complete picture.

At this very moment, there is someone being born and someone being buried, so should you be happy or sad? Can you be both at the same time?

Your individual perception is really like a piece of a giant puzzle that must be put together to get the truest picture. Sharing and learning through healthful communication, critical thinking, empathy, and comprehension are essential to knowing the truth that is reality—or the "big picture"—by engaging all of our prefrontal cortexes collectively (or at least that would be a great goal!).

And as we move into the future, what differentiates "virtual" reality from "actual" reality?

Ultimately it's the physical piece that differentiates the two—how what you are experiencing impacts your physical being. For example, when you're playing a virtual reality game, you are not physically injured if someone virtually shoots at you, even though you might hear it and see it, and maybe even feel a physical vibration through the virtual device.

The reason we use the word "reality" when it is "virtual" (or "not real") is because of how the experience affects you neurologically, mentally, and emotionally too, through your senses, just like the "real" physical world. If we can hear it and see it, then we perceive it as real. We need to engage all of our senses to determine if something is "actually" real, whether we can smell it, taste it, and physically feel it too, that indicates to our brain that it is part of our physical environment.

It can even be hard to distinguish a vivid dream or hallucination from reality when we aren't consciously aware of them, until we become conscious enough to use all of our senses. We might even pinch ourselves to see if we are in fact using all of our physical senses, or just dreaming.

Imagination and perception are similar but quite different, in that perception is how your brain puts all of your sensory information together unconsciously to formulate what is real, versus what is not. Imagination, on the other hand, is a conscious mental process to mimic sensations when they are not present. When someone is really good at mimicking reality in their mind, and even expressing it, we might say they have a vivid imagination.

For example, if I told you to imagine a dog barking, you could probably do it to some degree, and maybe even try to imitate it if I asked you to explain what it sounds like.

Perception, on the other hand, is when you actually hear a dog barking; that is, if your sense of hearing is not impaired. If you have hearing loss, you might perceive the bark differently than someone who has a keen sense of hearing. The one with hearing loss may not hear it at all, or might perceive it as a muffled noise, whereas the person with keen hearing might describe it as a piercing sound that almost gave them a headache.

The major difference between perception and imagination is that imagination only involves your mind and memory, while perception involves your mind, memory, and senses.

With perception, your memories act as a sort of filter when putting sensory information together that may result in a biased perception.

Perceptions of the same dog may be vastly different between two different people, with different knowledge, memories, and experiences. If one person has learned that dogs are violent and aggressive, or has even witnessed or experienced a traumatic dog attack, then the dog will immediately trigger their unconscious stress response as a perceived threat.

If the other person has owned and cared for many dogs, and has had far more positive experiences with dogs than negative experiences, then they will not immediately perceive the dog as a threat.

One will perceive the dog as a threat that triggers a stress response, while the other will not, and remains calm. The dog didn't change; it's just the human brains that are different, in how they respond to the same sensory stimulation, perceiving the same dog differently.

Similarly, if I believe something is a real threat to my physical health and safety, but you do not, how do we determine what's true and what isn't?

Who am I to tell you what to believe or what is real if we believe and experience different things in different ways?

I might start by presenting facts that can be proven using your own senses—maybe first something you can see, and then maybe something you can hear, or a combination of sight and sound. For better or worse, however, the added challenge these days is how easily recorded sights and sounds can be manipulated, altered, fabricated, and manufactured, that makes them nearly as hard to believe without additional proof or evidence—and most importantly, trust.

Ultimately, the most convincing proof is when you can experience something in first-person, physically for yourself, and even then you must trust your senses.

When you're trying to convince someone else that something you know is true, they first need to trust you and not perceive you as a threat. If they perceive you as a threat, then pretty much everything you say will be perceived as a threat and an attempt to manipulate them.

Never did I learn this more than while spending time alone with a beloved friend living with dementia, who is also blind.

While we were out sitting by the lake at her family's cabin one day, she looked at me in a panic and asked, "Why are they trying to kidnap me?"

I was completely startled and didn't know how to reply. I tried to calm her by saying, "You're OK. We're just at your family's lake cabin, and nobody is trying to kidnap you. We're out here by ourselves, but your kids all know where you are. They're just working, and we're safe. Everything is fine."

Then she asked one of the hardest questions I've ever been asked, "But how do you KNOW they're not trying to kidnap me?"

Never did I have a harder time coming up with words to help ease her mind. "Don't worry. Everything is fine. Your family knows where you are. You can trust me. We're only here until tomorrow." It all started to sound exactly like what someone who was trying to kidnap you would say, and I started to panic a little too, which I hoped wouldn't come across in my voice as a sign of trying to hide something from her.

I knew her unconscious stress response was telling her that she was in danger, which was especially powerful due to the dementia, impairing her prefrontal cortex, on top of her impaired vision. As frustrated as I felt, I had to remain calm in order to help calm her mind that required a sense of confidence and trust in me.

Rather than trying to rationalize with her (that would require engaging her impaired prefrontal cortex), I used something else that I knew would please her. I gave her one of her favorite things, a Hershey bar.

Thankfully, the chocolate gave her that little neurochemical boost she needed to help calm her amygdala (until I could give her a prescribed anti-anxiety medication to rebalance her neurochemistry).

This is why we enjoy "comfort foods" too—when we eat something that releases those feel-good neurochemicals associated with a pleasant memory or sense of comfort, safety, and happiness. Unfortunately, when we're conditioned to associate comfort with foods that are high in unhealthy fats and sugars, and other preservatives and artificial ingredients, we can develop unhealthy eating habits that have toxic effects on our neurology and physiology as well (nobody can survive on Hershey bars alone).

It sure felt like a sneaky thing to do, knowing how it would alter her emotional state like that. Using sweets and treats might work well in the short-term to influence someone to behave in a desired way, but can lead to long-term challenges when we are neurologically conditioned to rely on that sweet or treat to calm our unconscious stress response, especially when our impulse control is already inhibited.

This is also why humans in a heightened emotional state are especially vulnerable to emotional manipulation and irrational behavior, without the full powers of their prefrontal cortex to regulate emotions, control impulses, or think critically.

Similarly, trying to get someone else to believe you or see things from your perspective when they are full of emotion can be especially challenging, especially when they see you as a threat. When we don't trust people, it's our unconscious stress response that's running the show.

When we lack a sense of trust or confidence, stress can be a barrier to learning and understanding, or healing and resolve.

This is also the relationship between brain health, biases, and beliefs, based on the neurological balance between the amygdala and prefrontal cortex—influenced by who we trust and who we perceive as a threat.

Trust is really a means of lowering one's unconscious stress response in their amygdala to engage the higher functioning parts of their prefrontal cortex, including comprehension, critical thinking, problem solving, and empathy. When we experience stress without a sense of trust or confidence in what we are experiencing or being shown or told, we are less likely to comprehend and believe the information we are receiving.

Ultimately, we have to trust that the sights, sounds, tastes, smells, feelings, or other information and sensations (i.e., evidence) are real, and not just imaginary, false, or fabricated. This is really a self-defense mechanism, as part of our unconscious stress response to avoid being fooled or manipulated with a form of emotional mind control that could put us in jeopardy, into a situation that may be harmful to our health or well-being.

This is especially difficult these days when so much of what we see and hear (and even taste and smell) can be manufactured and manipulated in an attempt to influence our thoughts, feelings, perceptions, and behaviors. Stress is a deceptively effective motivator that keeps you coming back to make sure you haven't missed some critical resource or piece of information that could be detrimental to your health and happiness.

This is why human emotions are often so limiting, and why we need to be aware of them, and why we feel them.

To believe that we must all experience the same reality at the same time, to think and feel the same way at every moment, is one of the biggest barriers to our healing and well-being. To think that if one is down we must all be down, or if one is up we must all be up, is just too simplistic and unrealistic— because reality will always be a combination, with someone suffering while another is celebrating.

Social media complicates this even more by throwing everyone into the same pool at the same time, believing that everyone must think and feel the same at the same time. It creates this sense of angst and worry to miss a headline or story in order to not be perceived as out-of-touch, tone deaf, or insensitive. It's do or die, sink or swim, whether you like it or not.

Apps don't come with a "Surgeon General's Warning" with health instructions to use it wisely and healthfully, or how to reduce stress to engage our prefrontal cortex, to avoid being emotionally triggered and manipulated, to help put all of the pieces of our different life experiences and perspectives together into a complex collage that is the messy truth of reality.

Even when we consume the same information, our brains process it independently and differently than someone else's. Yet so often we expect everyone to process, feel, and react the same way, in order to feel like part of a collective group, when we often bond from a shared or similar fear or experience. When we don't know how the human brain works, it leaves us ignorant and vulnerable to often unnecessary and unhealthy conflict and confusion. Healthful communication, trust, and understanding are needed to help reduce stress to increase empathy, critical thinking, comprehension, impulse control, and emotional regulation—whether with a social group or between social groups.

This is part of the importance of raising awareness about

neurodiversity as well, to understand how different people process information and life experiences differently, and may respond to stress differently as well, when the amygdala is overactive or the prefrontal cortex is underdeveloped or inhibited.

When we realize that we don't all think or feel the same, much less at the same time, then life starts to make a little more sense, and can actually reduce stress.

One of the first questions to ask when it comes to changing behaviors is to understand your goal or intention, and how it makes you feel. Do you want to improve or achieve something to feel better? Will it improve your health, healing, acceptance, or resolve? Or is your goal to control a person or situation—if that's possible or healthful, for you and them?

Perception is indeed your reality. To say that your perception is not real, is to completely misunderstand what perception really is.

Your perception is like a puzzle that your brain pieces together with every sensation, that influences how you think about yourself, others, and the world around you.

Your greatest privilege and greatest pressure is how you perceive yourself, and how others perceive you. Your perception of me determines your level of trust and the influence I have over you, just as my perception of you determines my level of trust and the influence you have over me.

Do I perceive you as a team member or a competitor? Do I perceive you as my friend or my enemy?

Likewise, how do you perceive me?

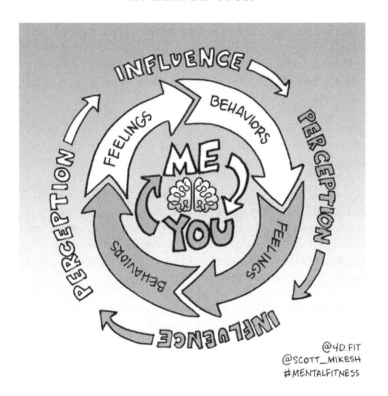

@4D.FIT
@SCOTT_MIKESH
#MENTALFITNESS

Due to how the brain works, the quickest way to make a friend is to treat someone like a friend, and the quickest way to make an enemy is to treat someone like an enemy.

If someone said they hate you, how would you feel and respond?

If someone said they love you, how would you feel and respond?

When someone perceives you as their enemy and treats you like their enemy, you are likely to feel and behave like their enemy. Likewise, if you perceive someone as your enemy and treat them like an enemy, they are likely to feel and behave like your enemy as well.

Similarly, perceptions can change over time—who you once perceived as your enemy may become your best friend, and who you once perceived as your best friend may become your worst enemy.

As animals, our stress response is often sensed by other animals as well (including other people). The stress hormone cortisol unconsciously alters our body chemistry without effort or awareness, increasing our heart rate, and inhibiting our emotional regulation and impulse control. This can trigger a slew of immediate unconscious physical responses like sweating and dry mouth, as well as body movements like flinching, scowling, staring, or other spontaneous gestures or comments that may be less-than-empathetic (since our stress response inhibits empathy as well).

Ultimately, it's how we treat each other and the emotions involved that either heighten or lower our unconscious stress response and either reinforce or resist an emotional bond. Your perception may be influenced by how someone looks, smells, sounds, or behaves, or what someone else said about them (that may or may not be true), or their association with others you either perceive as friends or enemies (as in "birds of a feather" or "guilty by association").

Those are factors in every relationship, really. How do you perceive them, and how do they perceive you?

Even more importantly, how do you perceive yourself?

When you have love for yourself, you feel less stressed when someone else doesn't love you, and you can maintain the power of your prefrontal cortex to maintain your own health and well-being. Similarly, by the powers of your prefrontal cortex, you are better able to love and forgive others, without feeling threatened by the possibility that they may not love you in return. This is the power of unconditional love, that does not feel threatened by the unloving sentiments or behaviors of another, and helps reduce your stress response to optimize your prefrontal cortex.

So much of our own attitude and self-perception is based on how others treat us, and what we interpret their responses, behaviors, and feedback to mean. Do we perceive ourselves as desirable, smart, successful, talented, liked, and appreciated? Or do we perceive ourselves as ugly, dumb, useless, talentless, disliked, and unappreciated?

You might feel things differently, see things differently, interpret things differently, taste things differently, smell things differently, or hear things differently based on any number of factors, whether due to your genetics or past experiences that have forged the neuropathways that exist in your brain, and no one else's.

These differences are truly exciting and should be shared and celebrated, not to be feared and criticized. They're just part of being the complex human beings we are, living in a complex natural world, with billions of life experiences happening all at once, with as many perspectives and perceptions of reality as there are people on the planet (mind blowing, I know!).

It's important to understand that diversity doesn't just exist between groups but also within the groups that we define as groups. There's not just one way of being, expressing, or experiencing life.

While there's a lot of pressure and attention on personal identity these days, what's often not discussed is the intense mental, emotional, and even physical processes involved when one's identity is not obvious and does not come easily. Self-discovery, self-love, and self-acceptance can take years of introspection and exploration, especially before someone feels comfortable enough to share their inner-most thoughts and feelings with the often quick-to-judge world.

For many, it can take decades to reach the point of self-love and confidence required for full public disclosure, if one is fortunate enough to achieve it in their lifetime. When we feel at odds with those around us, or forced to conform to rigid social standards or ways of being in order to feel respected and accepted by a group, the process of accepting and sharing our authentic selves becomes that much harder. Having to continuously open up, share, and even explain and defend yourself with everyone you meet can be extremely stressful and emotionally exhausting, especially when there is no end in sight.

It takes a lot of conscious energy and stress management to deal with social pressures and fear of rejection day-in and day-out. Stress not only affects your brain health and mental function, but also your physical health and function, including your digestive system, metabolic system, cardiovascular system, immune system, and reproductive system.

When we categorize, generalize, and stereotype people as homogenous monoliths within defined groups, we actually do more harm than good by perpetuating the very stereotypes, assumptions, and expectations that can be very limiting, unhealthy, and self-fulfilling in nature, since the human brain loves to be right (the power of reward) and does not like being wrong (the power of stress). We often go to great lengths to prove ourselves right, and to not be wrong (even if it means lying, manipulating, spinning, or fabricating facts and information—as a form of confirmation bias).

Since we don't all live the same life experiences, we need to make an effort to share and understand the experiences of each other, including different influences, environments, cultures, social and family dynamics, beliefs, body chemistry, and brains—to avoid the assumption that everyone does (or should) experience life in the same way.

Empathy is a function of the prefrontal cortex that provides an emotional experience based on another person's experience, when we attempt to think and feel as someone else does—not just as you would in their shoes, but as they do in their own— even when our own feelings and experiences may be vastly different. A great exercise for practicing empathy is to read stories about the feelings and life experiences of other people that allow you as the reader to experience their perspective and emotional experience.

Focusing on brain health and function reinforces why the practice of empathy as a function of the prefrontal cortex is so important to practice and understand, because empathy is inhibited when our unconscious stress response is triggered. It's not just because we're "bad," "uncooperative," or "unwilling," but because it's a very real and important neurological function of the human brain, that is not to be judged, but understood.

The conscious mental practice of empathy helps develop neuropathways beyond your own personal experience to consider the experiences of others using your imagination— including experiences of success, joy, and excitement as much as pain, loss, and sadness—thus developing a more complex and comprehensive perception of reality that allows you to learn new ways to understand and navigate life as well.

It's important to note that while the practice of empathy is considered to be healthful in many ways, empathy can also be harder and stress-inducing for those with an impaired or underdeveloped prefrontal cortex, or those who have a hard time regulating their emotions and maintaining emotional boundaries. The expectation that everyone can or should be able to practice and experience empathy in the same way, with the same healthful results and outcomes, is as unhealthful and unrealistic as expecting that everyone should be able to lift the same amount of weight, or run the same distance at the same speed.

Empathy is a neurological skill that requires practice, since it can often be difficult for different reasons, and may require support, instruction, or boundaries to practice in a healthful way.

We often associate empathy with caring and worry. Caring is considered a healthful emotional expression, while worry is considered an unhealthful emotional state. You can still care about another's well-being and experience without worrying about them, or taking on the stress and uncertainty of their situation that is outside of your control. Worry rarely has any health benefit, since it only sustains an unhealthy state of stress, with elevated levels of cortisol and no opportunity to resolve or remedy the situation. While it can be very difficult to not worry when we care, worry is also wasted energy.

If you are one who is highly sensitive and empathetic, who tends to feel the weight of the world and takes on the pain and problems of others, then your practice of empathy may require setting emotional boundaries to maintain a healthful mental state—to be able to care (by engaging your prefrontal cortex) without worry (without triggering your amygdala).

It's important to practice caring how others think and feel without worrying how others think and feel.

8 BIAS AND SELF-FULFILLING PROPHECY

Focusing on how the brain works can help you understand why you think, feel, and behave the way you do, and why others think, feel, and behave the ways they do, without bias or prejudice.

Just as it's important to understand the influences and impacts of stress, so must we be aware of the influences and impacts of bias. Related to your unconscious stress response, biases can have both healthful and unhealthful outcomes.

Bias is an inclination or prejudice for or against someone or something. Bias can be based on a sense of pleasure or familiarity, a preference for what or who you like or love, or a sense of safety and protection you feel. Bias can also be based on a sense of fear, discomfort, or dislike for someone or something you perceive as threatening, hurtful, or harmful, either from what you have personally experienced or witnessed, or what you've been taught or told.

When we are driven by our unconscious stress response, we inhibit our capacity to care and empathize. In addition, when we are desperate for support and understanding to help calm our stress response, we may become vulnerable to emotional manipulation and attack by those eager to exploit our pain for their own gain—by those who seek to increase their influence, power, and control of others.

When we experience an extreme sense of fear, distrust, or dislike, we can neurologically develop a powerful unconscious bias in our brain that inhibits the power of our prefrontal cortex—namely comprehension, critical thinking, problem solving, emotional regulation, impulse control, empathy, and compassion—that may result in violent or abusive behaviors.

Whether in humans or other animals, unconscious cues of prejudice perceived by one can trigger an unconscious stress response that can trigger aggressive or defensive behavior in the other or both, reinforcing the stress response in each. In psychology, this type of unconscious reinforcement is called a "self-fulfilling prophecy," when our own perceptions and stress response actually contribute to stressful outcomes that reinforce our stress response and bias. A self-reinforcing stress response can be a difficult pattern to break, that requires conscious effort to engage the prefrontal cortex to help mitigate and prevent our unconscious stress response.

When we challenge our biases and beliefs, a stress response known as "cognitive dissonance" can also occur, when beliefs that have been deeply forged into our neuropathways through repetition, reward, and reinforcement are challenged and forced to fire differently, that can cause discomfort and resistance. In a sense, it's almost like your prefrontal cortex and amygdala are firing at each other, with your amygdala being the most heavily armed with your primal unconscious stress response, that is difficult to disengage without a reward to power-up our prefrontal cortex. In just a few words, a friend can suddenly be perceived as a threat, and an enemy.

The vast differences in expectations and perceptions across different groups of people (that influence different neurological and physiological activity in the brain) contribute to all sorts of social, psychological, and behavioral conflicts and disparities.

Your amygdala is there for a reason—to protect you. As human beings trying to survive in an often uncertain world, our human brains just really want to be right and certain. Our human brains crave information to have a sense of knowledge, control, and certainty, to ease our unconscious stress response neurologically and physiologically by releasing those "feel good" neurochemicals like serotonin and dopamine. Therefore, your amygdala does not like to be wrong, since that would pose an even greater threat to your safety and well-being and trigger an unconscious stress response.

This unconscious neurological resistance to being wrong or incorrect is the basis of the phenomenon known as "confirmation bias," when we unconsciously seek information that validates our unconscious emotions and stress response, that feels better than consciously challenging them. For this reason, we may unconsciously fill in the gaps of what we don't know with ideas of what might be, to achieve a sense of certainty.

When we only accept information that does not trigger our unconscious stress response, we limit our understanding and opportunity to achieve healthful outcomes as well.

For example, when we limit our understanding of mental health conditions to only those symptoms that do not threaten anyone other than the person experiencing the mental health condition, then we overlook, disregard, shame, judge, and stigmatize symptoms like anger, aggression, hostility, and violence associated with various mental and neurochemical conditions, due to our own unconscious bias, fear, and stress response that inhibits our ability to empathize and comprehend.

This is part of the stigma that surrounds mental healthcare—when different brain health conditions have different symptoms that we fear and stigmatize.

We often depict the villain or killer as a "sociopath" or "psycho" in media and movies, even though the vast majority of people with mental illnesses are not killers or villains, and are even law-abiding citizens with families, jobs, and people who love them.

Is the quiet, unkempt, or socially awkward person you work with or live next to really scary and creepy, or are they living with a neurological difference or mental health condition that may or may not be diagnosed or healthfully managed?

The moment someone behaves in a way that triggers our unconscious stress response, we judge them as inappropriate, shameful, or immoral, and our sense of empathy and compassion goes right out the window.

In this day and age, we would never allow someone to be publicly shamed for having a physical illness or disability, but unfortunately, our society has not yet evolved to the point of having empathy or understanding for someone with a mental health condition or neurological difference.

We don't yet publicly cheer people on who are struggling with a mental illness the way we cheer people on who are struggling with a physical illness, and we don't yet champion early detection, diagnosis, treatment, and prevention of brain health conditions to the degree that we champion efforts for physical health conditions.

Out of fear, we often resort to separation, segregation, and isolation as a "quick fix"—the idea being that if we stay away from those we perceive as a threat, who trigger our unconscious stress response, then we will maintain a sense of safety that allows us to feel and do our best by calming our amygdala and optimizing our prefrontal cortex. To reduce our unconscious stress response, we live in separate houses, have different spaces to practice different religions, have different work spaces and schools for different kinds of people, and have invisible borders that keep different groups of people apart.

I don't mean to imply what is right or wrong, but rather what is and why—in order to navigate this complex world in the healthiest way possible, for everyone.

While separation and segregation might help avoid stressful situations with a greater sense of safety and protection by avoiding the stress of dealing with differences, it can also contribute to fear and biases as well. Avoidance does little to help us heal or avoid the formation of biases, or our ability to develop more healthful perceptions and more resilient mental practices when we experience stress or a perceived threat.

Since unconscious biases are neurological in nature, they must also be treated and healed as such through some form of exposure therapy that often requires the support of a licensed therapist. By slowly exposing the person to the stressful stimulus, bit by bit, they can gradually retrain their brain by repeating and reinforcing new neuropathways in a less stressed state, to ultimately reduce their unconscious stress response and engage their prefrontal cortex.

9 PAIN IS A SIGNAL NOT TO IGNORE

When it comes to fitness practices, we often confuse pain and discomfort by saying, "No pain no gain!"

For the sake of both your mental and physical well-being, it's important to understand and differentiate the neurological signals of pain and discomfort to respond to each in the most healthful way.

Discomfort is a neurological signal—whether an unpleasant site, sound, taste, smell, thought, or feeling—that indicates you need to change, shift, or rebalance something before it causes harm or damage. For example, when you sit in an uncomfortable chair, your sense of discomfort is an indicator that an adjustment is needed before it causes you more harm or pain. You might be able to tolerate staying in that uncomfortable position for a few minutes or even a few hours, but the longer you remain in that state or position the more likely it will lead to more serious harm or damage. Remaining in an uncomfortable position may even require conscious effort to regulate and reduce your unconscious stress response (that is often a mental practice associated with Buddhist monks).

Pain, on the other hand, is a neurological signal that indicates harm or damage is either happening at that moment or has happened, and must be rectified immediately by stopping, recovering, or seeking care. You don't remain seated on a scorching hot chair for more than a split second when your pain signal tells you, "DO NOT SIT HERE!" If you ignore or tolerate your pain signal and remain seated to "work through the pain," you will no doubt get seriously burned and cause further harm to your system.

It's not just your physical anatomy that senses pain or illness either, and it's not just physical illness, imbalance, or injury that can threaten your health and well-being. It's just as important (if not more) to be aware of how you feel mentally and emotionally as well as physically, to understand what your brain and body are trying to tell you when something isn't quite right. Maybe it's an ache or a pain, or a general sense of dread or hopelessness. Maybe it's a rush of emotions that make you feel like you can't breathe, or a mix of thoughts and feelings that make your head feel like it's about to pop off.

Neurologically, pain is a signal that something needs to heal, recover, or should be removed and avoided completely.

Growth and adaptation are not the result of pain but rather the result of noticing it and responding accordingly.

Therefore, pain is neither a sign of strength nor a sign of weakness, but rather a neurological signal—whether from stress, pressure, illness, imbalance, or injury—that requires immediate care and attention. Pain is a signal that a condition needs to be noticed and cared for in order to heal and recover, not ignored or sustained, especially when there is nothing to be gained other than more pain and injury.

There is no health benefit to enduring pain when it prolongs the problem and delays proper care, treatment, healing, recovery, and prevention. Not taking your pain seriously can lead to serious illness, injury, or imbalance that makes the pain worse, and doesn't make you stronger.

Contrary to the old saying "no pain, no gain" (that should really say "no challenge, no gain" to be more accurate, but doesn't rhyme as well) you can absolutely gain without pain, and should! The process may be challenging and uncomfortable, but need not be painful, that's important to differentiate as well.

Fitness programs are never a substitute for healing and recovery, which is why prior to beginning any fitness program—whether physical or mental—you should consult your physician or therapist to ensure that you are ready and able to do the physical and mental exercises involved, depending on your fitness goals and needs.

The same basic neurological principles apply for exercising and developing your brain and body, with the first step being neurological balance and stability. When it comes to optimizing and improving performance either mentally or physically, you first need to develop and strengthen your functional foundation that is your neurological system.

Healthful fitness practices begin by practicing balance, to strengthen your neurological foundation on which everything else is built—to maintain healthful form and function. This is also why an underdeveloped foundation can result in imbalance or injury, when more work and pressure is demanded than we are prepared to perform.

An ounce of prevention through awareness and education really is worth a pound of cure.

When you work your muscles in a way that demands more work than they're used to, the muscle fibers tear in microscopic ways that triggers a physiological response by releasing amino acids to help them heal. It's this build-up of acid that makes your muscles feel sore and uncomfortable, that we learn to differentiate from the pain of an injury.

It's important to differentiate these neurological sensations in order to know your limits to prevent injury, both mentally and physically.

It's actually the time between workouts (mentally or physically) when growth and adaptation take place, not during the workout itself, since your brain and body need time to rest, repair, and heal, to grow and prepare for next time.

10 CHANGE, GRIEF, AND ADAPTATION

It's important to know that not every change is healthful, and there's a healthful reason why your unconscious stress response is triggered by your amygdala when you feel forced to change without a choice or an immediate benefit. That's the way every human brain works, in defense against potential threats to our health and well-being.

What can get in our way is when we confuse the word "acceptance" with approval, endorsement, or resignation. For example, accepting that you have cancer that requires treatment is neither endorsing cancer nor resigning to it. Acceptance is simply the mental state of accepting what is in order to reduce our unconscious stress response by activating the powers of our prefrontal cortex. This process requires a neurological shift that can be a painful process, depending on the severity and emotional intensity of the change.

Our stress response has good intention. The amygdala unconsciously jumps into action in order to protect us from harm, to get us to a place where we feel safe and secure again. Our unconscious response is also based on neurological signals transmitted unconsciously through our autonomic nervous system before our conscious mind receives them or has a chance to comprehend and understand the situation.

When something is a threat to our own life or well-being, or the life and well-being of someone we love (who stimulates that sense of safety and security for us), it makes sense why we would try to control, cage, contain, prevent, cure, or otherwise stop that threat from causing us pain, harm, or damage. This is how our conscious mind rationalizes and reinforces our unconscious stress response.

When we choose to be curious rather than controlling, however, we naturally reduce our unconscious stress response by calming the amygdala and engaging our prefrontal cortex to achieve a sense of acceptance that drives comprehension, critical thinking, empathy, and problem solving.

So please be gentle with yourself (and others) when dealing with grief, trauma, or any significant change that alters your sense of safety and security (whether you understand it or not), as you search for a sense of hope to help reduce your stress response, and allow neurological healing and homeostasis to take its place.

Common ways to reduce the unconscious stress response in humans include raising awareness of the rewards and benefits of a change, or giving people a choice between multiple options. Both of these practices stimulate a greater sense (or perception) of control, and reduce our unconscious stress response.

Consider the difference between being forced to leave your home on a moment's notice with no other choice, versus the choice to sell and make a profit or moving into your dream home with plenty of time to plan and prepare.

Both are types of "change," but one comes with more stress

and fewer benefits than the other. When we have little time, power, control, influence, benefits, or options, the change is much more challenging to navigate physically, mentally, and emotionally due to the level of our unconscious stress response that is trying to protect us.

When talking about "change," it's important to differentiate between healthful (that promotes health) versus unhealthful (that poses a risk) change, and whether it involves adaptation (a healthful process to thrive) or conformity (a stress-inducing demand to comply).

There's a neurological reason why it's easier to embrace change when there's an obvious and immediate benefit or reward, and why it's much harder when the change we face is difficult, doesn't feel good, or has no obvious or immediate benefit.

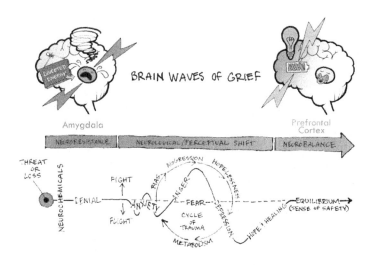

This neurological process is related to the process we call "grief"—when what used to stimulate pleasure no longer does, as your brain works to adapt to the change of this new reality. Your brain is seeking a sense of reward, safety, and comfort again—that can result in waves of denial, bargaining, fear, anger, anxiety, and depression. The grieving process requires a sense of hope in order to reduce your unconscious stress response and activate your prefrontal cortex, as your neuropathways adjust to a state of comprehension, emotional regulation, critical thinking, and acceptance.

Grief can happen when something that makes you feel safe, content, loved, joyful, or happy changes or goes away.

Freeing ourselves from those controlling forces and limitations that hold us back—to feel and do our best, to make honest and healthful choices, to be our honest and authentic selves —is what empowerment is all about.

The neurological conundrum is that "change" often involves imposing stress or pressure to force an outcome that often results in an unconscious stress response (i.e., triggering the amygdala, producing excess cortisol, reacting with resistance, etc.) that can contribute to less healthful outcomes. When we're more focused on controlling outcomes than promoting individual empowerment, we're also less focused on understanding and acceptance.

As the saying goes, "If you love it, set it free."

Growth happens when the weight is lifted and we're allowed to develop with healthful guidance and support, without the imposing stress or restrictive pressures of control.

Empowerment is really about having faith and trust in ourselves and each other to do the healthful thing—even when that means learning from our mistakes, to accept what we can and can't control. When something is "out of control" or outside of your control, it can feel risky and dangerous, that again triggers your unconscious stress response.

Of course sometimes controls are necessary to maintain order, to feel safe when we're afraid. Just as important in those moments of fear, is to understand WHY we feel stress or react with resistance, and WHY it's so hard to feel and do our best, when our sense of freedom is limited or restricted.

When you find yourself irritated, worried, or anxious about a conflict or confrontation (with a flush face, racing heart, and breathing hard), practice taking deep controlled breaths to soothe your sympathetic nervous system and lower your unconscious stress response. Inhale slowly and deeply for approximately four seconds, hold it for approximately four seconds, and then exhale slowly and deeply for approximately four seconds, focusing on your breath the entire time. Repeat that breathing pattern to reduce your stress response until you feel a more balanced sense of mental and emotional stability to engage your prefrontal cortex.

Ask yourself, "What can I do in this moment to deescalate the situation?"

When you approach a conflict with an attitude of curiosity and empowerment, by accepting and respecting how the human brain works (including your own), you can help lower the stress level to increase comprehension and improve communications, to replace resistance with cooperation, to achieve a more healthful outcome.

When you're not allowed to challenge or ask questions about a change or loss, your unconscious stress response can be further triggered as a warning sign.

When we're forced to change (e.g., with a death, job loss, or divorce), challenging and questioning the change can be done in a healthful way that allows us to find growth and meaning in it, to support our health, healing, and resilience. Expecting immediate acceptance of change or loss, without allowing it to be challenged or questioned (by the unconscious stress response of the one being challenged or questioned), only prevents this critical neurological step in the grieving process, that ultimately allows us to learn, heal, and grow by reaching a more balanced state of trust, hope, comprehension, and acceptance.

It's simply not enough (nor healthy or effective) to tell people "what" to do, think, or believe, especially without considering "why" we do, think, or believe what we do—how thoughts, feelings, perceptions, and attitudes are formed physiologically, and how they influence our choices, actions, habits, and behaviors—that ultimately impact our health, success, and well-being.

Whether healthful or unhealthful, navigating change is not easy, and takes effort. We often use the analogy of "digging ourselves into a hole" when it seems our reaction to a stressful situation makes things worse (thanks to our unconscious stress response). To climb out of that hole, we must first look up, with the hope that there is a way out, to activate our prefrontal cortex.

When we're in that pit of despair, we often lose hope, and quite literally keep looking and feeling down (i.e., stress) because we don't believe there's a reason to look up. We sometimes get so low that we don't want to move, or wish we were out of sight and out of reach from whatever is causing us pain.

Sometimes we try to help others with what we consider "advice," but just make things worse by being smug, condescending, or even shameful with comments like...

"You really need to stop doing that to yourself and snap out of it."

"I wish you would open your eyes and see how good things really are."

"You just have to stop feeling sorry for yourself and try harder!"

As if our pain is a choice? As if we're not trying hard enough? As if we can't see the situation clearly?

What we often fail to realize is how often our neurological feelings and sensations are not something we can control, but must be felt, acknowledged, and understood, not just ignored or swept under the rug. Your feelings could be related to a situation in your life as much as a lack of sleep, nutrition, or oxygen, or a symptom of a more serious health condition or neurochemical imbalance, or all of the above.

For things to change, you must first feel what you feel, to understand why, to perceive the possibility that things can change for the better, to believe in your healing ability and adaptability, to think about things differently—that requires a sense of hope or optimism to reduce your unconscious stress response and activate your prefrontal cortex.

Mental fitness practices focus on building that sense of hope, motivation, and support you need, to navigate whatever stress and change come your way, to achieve healthful outcomes and adapt in a way that helps you thrive!

11 CRAPPINESS CAN LEAD TO HAPPINESS

Life might be full of crappy moments, but happiness can also grow from those crappy moments like fertilizer.

As I like to say, the grass might seem greener on the other side because there's more sh*t over there (it's just hard to smell until you're standing in it).

Since happiness is a neurological response, it can either be fleeting and difficult to find, or more attainable and easier to maintain, depending on how you experience and define the feeling of happiness.

It's important to realize that your body is constantly trying to rebalance itself to a point of homeostasis, which is why those extreme feelings of high and low will come and go, relatively speaking. For some, homeostasis may be higher or lower levels of certain neurochemicals, which is why it's important to understand what you feel and why, to determine if you may need more support, therapeutic services, or supplements to sustain a more healthful balance or homeostasis.

This rebalancing is what contributes to your ability to acclimate and adapt, to maintain neurological balance in different situations.

If you define "happiness" as that momentary euphoric rush of pure bliss and excitement, void of any stress, pain, or problems that naturally happen along the way, then this type of happiness will not only be difficult to find but also impossible to maintain. When you do achieve that euphoric rush, the flood of "feel good" neurochemicals quickly dissipates as your neurochemistry naturally rebalances toward homeostasis again.

When those "feel good" neurochemicals temporarily mask pain or discomfort, we may be more inclined to seek other experiences (or chemicals) to feel that neurochemical rush again. Attempts to mimic those happy feelings to mask pain or discomfort are just as short-lived, and might lead to risky behaviors or chemical abuse as your brain and body continue to rebalance and adapt each time, requiring more and more to achieve that neurochemical rush (if achievable at all). This is essentially the neurochemical process behind addiction.

On the other hand, if you define "happiness" as a state of contentment, even when you might be managing stress, pain, or problems that prevent you from feeling a state of euphoria, then this is a more healthful, achievable, and sustainable state, since it's not the result of a neurochemical rush but rather the result of a balanced neurochemical state. This is, in part, why the practice of gratitude is so powerful when it comes to calming your amygdala by engaging your prefrontal cortex, by focusing on what's already in your life that you feel grateful for, to help you rebalance your neurochemistry with a sense of contentment—that might provide the sense of happiness you seek.

For this reason, comparison is often considered the thief of happiness. Rather than focusing on what you do have and how to make the most of it (by engaging your prefrontal cortex), comparison influences your thinking (by triggering your unconscious stress response) to perceive happiness as being what others have and you don't, thereby making you feel that you are missing out or don't have what it takes.

It's the disappointment we feel when expectations are not met that causes a stress response and triggers a sudden crash of neurochemicals that causes that sense of depression and unhappiness.

Setting achievable goals and realistic expectations, however, can help maintain a more balanced and sustainable neurochemical state. This is what can make the pursuit of happiness in itself so motivating and exhilarating, with anticipation of the reward, by sustaining those neurochemicals associated with happiness.

As it's often said, happiness is not a destination but the journey itself, that allows you to feel those good feelings at different points along the way, to maintain your sense of excitement and motivation to continue your journey.

Pursuing happiness as your motivation can actually be rewarding in itself, with the excitement we feel from the anticipation! This is the benefit of practicing delayed gratification and setting realistic achievable goals.

Similarly, this is what happens with physical exercise, when muscles adapt to the work that's demanded of them and stop building when repeating the same amount and type of work (that we call conditioning). When you want to build muscle, you must change the amount of weight and types of exercises you do to induce muscle confusion, thereby challenging your muscle tissue to heal, grow, and adapt.

Much like your muscles, your brain is constantly trying to adapt to the work that's demanded of it, that is also a form of conditioning

It's also important to understand the process of conditioning and adaptation to ensure you condition and adapt in healthful ways. For example, if you adapt to a stressful environment, then you may have a harder time navigating a low-stress environment, and may seek stressful situations that feel more comfortable and familiar. If you have adapt to a low-stress environment, then you may find it more difficult to navigate a high-stress environment, and may seek lower stress environments that feel more comfortable and familiar. The key is really to find the right balance of challenge and adaption to achieve the healthiest outcomes.

Similar to physical exercise, a healthful state is not necessarily repeating the same work or exercises, but challenging your system to readapt, to promote growth, flexibility, and adaptability. This is why lifelong learning is so important, to challenge yourself with new ideas, creative projects, or games to stimulate your brain in new ways, to reinforce growth and adaptability.

Due to how your unconscious stress response works, often times the path to true happiness is to first want happiness for others, thereby reducing our need to compare and compete, freeing ourselves to feel grateful for what we have as well. When we are not able to feel happiness for others (due to our unconscious stress response), we may have a harder time feeling happy for ourselves as well, since our unconscious stress response remains in an active state, fueled by the threat of comparison and competition, .

As is often said, we reap what we so. In other words, what we seek is what we eventually find. When we're focused on problems and expend our energy on worrying and consuming bad news (driven by our unconscious stress response), then that is what we'll find, reinforce, and cultivate.

In a sense, you can practice turning your fear, pain, and discomfort into fertilizer by engaging your prefrontal cortex to learn, adapt, and grow. Think of an experience that was painful, scary, or embarrassing for you. While the memory might be painful or unpleasant to think about, did you learn something from it? Did you learn what to avoid or how to approach similar situations in a more productive or healthful way?

This is also why it's important to reassess your goals and expectations at varying points in your journey too, when your system rebalances itself back to homeostasis, as you adapt and acclimate.

12 TRAUMA, TRIGGERS, AND ABUSE

Do you struggle with self-doubt, insecurities, negative self-talk, shame, or guilt? Do you feel a lack of confidence and motivation, or a general fear of not being liked, accepted, or good enough?

If you answer "yes" to any or all of the above, you are normal and not alone!

Some of those feelings may be the result of very stressful and traumatic lived experiences, or the result of mental, emotional, or physical abuses.

Whether with family, friends, coworkers, or sexual partners, what makes abuse even harder to identify is when abusive behaviors become normalized from how we were raised, to what society teaches us, to what we see in media, to what we've experienced in past relationships that come to be expected and accepted as "normal" behaviors. In a sense, we become acclimated or desensitized by repeated exposure as an unhealthy form of neurological adaptation (i.e., trauma bonding).

While it's much easier to see the physical signs of physical abuse, the signs of mental and emotional abuse can be much harder to spot and identify, and therefore much harder to treat and heal. Without physical evidence or visual clues, the effects of mental and emotional trauma and abuse can fester and manifest in our thoughts, feelings, and behaviors—including abusive behaviors toward others.

It can be especially difficult to identify mental and emotional abuse when power dynamics are involved—including demands and expectations, coercion and intimidation, codependence and threats of abandonment—that put extra pressure on the one experiencing abuse to hide or otherwise feel shame or guilt for the pain they feel.

The one experiencing abuse may also be shamed for "allowing" the abuse to occur, especially by those who are emotionally connected to the one behaving abusively.

This is due to how the brain works. We have a harder time comprehending how someone we perceive as "good" could do something "bad," just as we can have difficulty comprehending (or trusting) how someone we perceive as "bad" could do something "good." The conflict of emotionally-driven information triggers an unconscious stress response in the brain, activating the amygdala and inhibiting the powers of the prefrontal cortex, including critical thinking, comprehension, emotional regulation, and empathy.

It's important to note that being victimized and traumatized by mental and emotional abuse is not a sign of weakness, ignorance, gullibility, fragility, or vulnerability. The ability to spot and identify mental and emotional abuse when it is happening to you or someone else is actually a sign of emotional strength and healthful awareness.

Even when subtle and gradual, abuse is what abuse does.

When what you are experiencing physically, mentally, or emotionally becomes detrimental to your health and well-being by manifesting in unhealthy thoughts, feelings, and behaviors—or limiting your ability to heal and receive proper care—then abuse it is.

The toxic effects of abuse include learning and repeating abusive behaviors as a coping mechanism, when we find power and comfort in abusing others the way we were abused, by releasing a bit of adrenaline and dopamine that helps soothe our unconscious stress response. It's critical to recognize, identify, and treat trauma not only to heal it but also to prevent it from spreading to others—much like an emotional virus, spreading from one person to another.

Mental and emotional abuses may include:

- Jealousy of your success, friendships, and relationships (even family members)
- Gaslighting or lying about events to fit a false self-serving narrative (to shame or confuse you)
- Blaming you for their actions or what's wrong in their life
- Ignoring and disrespecting your personal boundaries
- Humiliating or berating you in public or in private
- Threatening to hurt themselves because of you
- Shaming you for your feelings so you won't have the courage to talk to others about their abuse
- Repeatedly being extra sweet and loving after the abuse (until it happens again)
- Using your love for them to control you
- Trying to make you feel ashamed, guilty, or afraid
- Putting their needs and feelings above yours, as the only ones that matter in the relationship

You may feel constantly judged and criticized when you are the target of abuse, like nothing you say or do is ever good enough. The person abusing you may accuse you of being incapable or distrustful, with no respect or compassion for you or your feelings. They might monitor your location or spy on you in an attempt to intimidate and control your daily life (even online).

Gaslighting is a toxic form of mental abuse that attempts to push your stress level and emotions to the breaking point, by rejecting what you say and twisting your words until you get so frustrated, confused, and exhausted that you fight, flee, or freeze—by emotionally erupting, agreeing in defeat, or complying with their demands.

People who gaslight you WANT you to react in an unhealthy stressed-out way, in order to get you to do or say what they want, that may not be what you would otherwise say or do in a healthy mental state. You might get angry, violent, or confused, or take risks you wouldn't otherwise take, so they can then blame and shame you for your stress response, as a form of confirmation bias to prove themselves right.

This form of emotional abuse has unfortunately been normalized under the guise of "debate," especially online. Gaslighting is especially tricky since unconscious biases are used and manipulated by the one perpetrating the abuse to twist and confuse our perception of the situation. The major difference being that healthy debate actually requires listening and critical thinking (powered by the prefrontal cortex), not just beating one's chest until someone surrenders (powered by the amygdala).

Gaslighting is a serious form of emotional abuse that must be recognized and understood in order to provide proper care and prevention.

Whether the form of abuse is mental or emotional (attacking your thoughts and feelings), or physical (attacking your body), any form of abuse can put your mental and physical health at risk, since cortisol can wreak havoc on your brain and body, and have devastating neurological effects on your thoughts, feelings, and behaviors.

Remember that you DO have the right to set personal boundaries and choose who you allow into your personal space—physically, mentally, and emotionally—that must be respected. Anyone who does not respect your thoughts, feelings, mental health, physical health, or personal boundaries does not respect you, and does not deserve your time and attention.

As a human being, you have every right to protect your physical and mental health by blocking toxicity, not only from social media, but in your life in general. In doing so, you also give the person or people behaving in abusive ways the time and space they need to heal too. It's up to you to decide if, when, or how they may be allowed back into your personal space, with your consent, once they have taken accountability for their own health, healing, and recovery.

Unlike physical pain and injury, severe mental pain and emotional trauma can take much longer to heal than physical wounds, due to their invisibly neurological nature as well. Proper care and healing is too often not received when emotional trauma is ignored, unrecognized, and untreated, with severe health consequences that can last a lifetime.

It's important to remember that the traumatic experience and toxic effects of abuse apply to every human being, and not just one particular group or type of person. Statistically speaking, we are often abused most by the people we love the most, making the mental and emotional abuse that much more painful and harder to recognize and heal, when we also want to protect the person who is abusing us, who at other times makes us feel safe and secure.

When it comes to mental abuse, it can become increasingly difficult to distinguish the "abused" from the "abuser" since our natural response to abusive behaviors may be to fight back in abusive ways, to regain a sense of power and control of the situation by using similar tactics—fighting fire with fire. Without awareness or accountability, it can become a battle of wits between people who each believe they are the victim of the abuse. For this reason, it's more healthful to not label people and instead identify the specific behaviors as abusive and unhealthy, in an effort to help heal all involved, who have likely all been abused and traumatized in some way.

All parties involved may require counseling and therapy to distinguish the source of their pain, the damaging effects of abuse, and ways to heal themselves and their relationship (if their relationship is healthy enough to recover). Therefore, it's often less helpful or healthful to place blame and labels, and more helpful and healthful to identify the unhealthy influences, feelings, and behaviors that require awareness, care, and healing.

I don't say this as a counselor or therapist, but to advocate for the critical importance of clinical counseling and therapy.

When it comes to behavior change, it's really not about trying to forcibly control behaviors or forcibly change minds through threats or intimidation (that often lead to further conflict or temporary conformity), but rather understanding minds by focusing on healthful function, influence, and outcomes.

It's not about being right or morally superior, but rather understanding what's hard to understand, when others have beliefs or behaviors different from your own, especially when their beliefs or behaviors cause harm to themselves or others.

Due to the unconscious nature of your stress response and its connection to long-term memory, however, it takes many more safe and friendly exposures (known as exposure therapy) to undo the neurological effects created by stresses and threats.

If you are attacked by a dog as a child before you develop positive memories and knowledge about dogs, the traumatic experience may be more likely to trigger a general fear of dogs that may require exposure therapy to heal those traumatic long-term memories that unconsciously trigger your stress response (a.k.a. unconscious bias).

Conversely, if you are attacked by a dog as an adult after years of positive experiences and knowledge of how to behave with dogs, understanding why dogs behave the way they do, you may be far less likely to develop the same level of emotional trauma as you would have as a child.

Because of your vast positive experiences with dogs and the healthful memories you have developed, you may perceive the attack as an exception rather than the rule. In a way, your lived experiences and collection of positive memories counteract your unconscious stress response from that singular attack. While you may be more cautious around that particular kind of dog, you are probably less likely to develop a general fear of dogs as an adult, as you may have as a child, with fewer memories and experiences to counteract the trauma.

As humans, we tend to be better at reaction than prevention—that is, reacting to a condition or situation rather than preventing it—in part, because we can't predict the future, and one of our primary motivators is our reactive stress response.

Since your amygdala receives neurological signals before your prefrontal cortex, most of your choices and behaviors are emotionally driven unconsciously. When we say "trust your gut" or "follow your heart," what we're really saying is follow your emotions. We usually then try to rationalize them after the fact, since that's how the brain works—with the amygdala receiving signals first, followed by the prefrontal cortex (once the amygdala calms down). The real key to practicing proactive, preventive, healthful behaviors is to be emotionally aware of what's influencing your emotions neurologically.

When we are reactively driven by stress (even in the habit of procrastination), we don't feel motivated until a problem occurs, often until something is hurt or broken—when it's much harder to heal and fix.

When we focus on prevention, then the problem itself need not occur to maintain our purpose and motivation. Rather, we switch from being reactive to proactive, from being driven by fear and pain to being driven by hope and healing, from being driven by our unconscious stress response (with cortisol and adrenaline) to being driven by critical thinking and problem solving, that helps regulate our emotions, heart rate, metabolism, and impulse control by engaging the prefrontal cortex (with the release of related neurochemicals).

It's much more effective and efficient to focus on such things as fitness, safety, and prevention to avoid the difficult, costly, and time-consuming process of recovery.

Unfortunately, since we as humans will never know what we don't know until it slaps us in the face, we tend to believe that we have better solutions when all we know is what we know, without knowing it all.

This is similar to the difference in how it feels to be the one being criticized (OUCH!) compared to how it feels to criticize someone else (take THAT!).

Of course it feels very different when we are the one with the power and influence than the one who is powerless. It's also hard to empathize and see things from another's perspective when we're in a stressed "us vs. them" state, especially when stress feels empowering with that intoxicating rush of adrenaline.

Whoever you are, there is someone out there who wants you to feel bad about yourself, for being who you are, because you challenge their thoughts and feelings that triggers their stress response in some way—whether it's from something you did or said to them directly, or based on what you represent as a person, that triggers their unconscious bias.

When someone gets an adrenaline rush from making you feel bad, they might even try to build you up at first, by becoming your friend, to influence and manipulate your feelings in a way that makes you feel you have to seek their approval, forgiveness, or validation—with a rewarding rush of dopamine when you do—that helps them feel better about themselves. This is also why someone who wants you to feel bad may even get more enraged, when their efforts fail and backfire—when you don't feel bad or feel the need to seek their approval, forgiveness, or validation.

This type of emotional abuse and manipulation is considered emotional grooming. They might try to limit your ability to be your free and authentic self because you trigger their stress response by challenging their unconscious biases, maybe even making them aware of things they don't like about themselves.

When one amygdala is triggered, there is nothing it wants more than to find something to fight or flee—which is what leads to confirmation bias—to find something or someone to fight to prove their stress response right, that gives them a brief rush of dopamine that momentarily calms their stress response (the sweet taste of victory!).

Until we heal our trauma and triggers, this repeated pattern of triggers and trauma will continue.

In order to heal and prevent abusive behaviors, mental and emotional abuses must be taken as seriously as physical and sexual abuses—from which the mental and emotional trauma can be the most damaging and lasting injury as well—since the neurological scars of emotional trauma last a lifetime, and emotions influence our behaviors.

It's important to understand the kinds and signs of abuse and other emotional challenges that may be a byproduct of more general fears and feelings that develop from a combination of internal and external influences, including how you were raised, the environment in which you lived, what you've been taught and told, your diet and body chemistry, or any combination.

It's important to be aware of how you think and feel, along with how your brain and body work, so you can tell when you need extra care, healing, exercise, or support.

As a neurological defense system, your amygdala is also linked to your long-term memory to support your survival by remembering the threats that you experience, to fight or avoid even faster next time—what we otherwise identify as biases, fears, and phobias.

Highly stressful or traumatic episodes (whether lived first-person or witnessed third-person) are quickly embedded in your brain like a neurochemical burn—that can lead to mental health conditions such as emotional triggers, anxiety, depression, and even PTSD (Post-Traumatic Stress Disorder).

When your stress response overwhelms your system, you might even experience a state of *shock*, with symptoms including shortness of breath, a severe drop in blood pressure, loss of consciousness, and even short-term memory loss. This "overload" response is considered a form of instinctual self-defense, since it momentarily disengages your prefrontal cortex to prevent conscious awareness of the traumatic event.

That said, even though your conscious mind may be disengaged to prevent conscious awareness of a traumatic experience, that doesn't mean the traumatic episode didn't have an impact on your brain, body, and neurology. To the contrary, the impact of trauma on your brain and body (including your ANS and amygdala) is still very real. Even though you may not be consciously aware, you may experience physical or mental health symptoms, either shortly after the event, or even years later.

When I was around the age of five, my family was in a horrific car accident that nearly killed us all. My brother was four and my sister was around eight.

Moments after our mom picked us up from daycare, we were broadsided by a speeding car that was racing through the otherwise quiet neighborhood. We were one block away from our daycare and five blocks away from our house.

Mom was crushed by the steering wheel, breaking several of her ribs and puncturing her lung. My sister was in the back seat and suffered the most serious injuries. Her face smashed through the window on one side and her leg smashed through the other. She had lacerations across her face that required reconstructive surgery and broke her femur bone in two places (that later had to be re-broken and reset since it didn't heal correctly the first time).

Miraculously, my brother and I were thrown under the dashboard and sustained only minor bumps and bruises.

To this day, I have no conscious memory of the accident. The firefighters who were first on the scene removed my brother and me from the wreckage. I only know that from pictures and stories that made it into the news.

All I remember was "waking up" in a wheelchair in the

hospital emergency room, watching cartoons. It took me a while to regain full consciousness, and I still remember that moment in the hospital like it was yesterday, burned into my long-term neurochemical memory. My vision was blurred and my head felt heavy. I was drooling on myself but couldn't help it. I was later told that I had been in a state of shock, unable to walk or talk for hours. I felt like I'd been drugged, with no conscious memory of the accident or how I got to the hospital.

I now realize that whatever I saw or heard during the accident was too much for my young brain to take, and it's buried somewhere deep in my unconscious brain. It makes me thankful for the stress response we have, that prevented that horrific bloody memory from haunting my dreams and consciousness. I can't imagine having to relive those painful memories over and over again, though I'm sure the experience impacted my mental health in some unknown way, that likely contributed to the anxiety I've struggled with most my life as well.

Empowering yourself to make your mental health a priority begins by helping you understand, accept, and care for your brain in healthful ways, including awareness of the complex effects of trauma and abuses, the importance of mental healthcare and healing, and the power of mental fitness practices.

13 TOXICITY OF "US VS. THEM"

As a species, we naturally gravitate toward those who stimulate a sense of trust and safety (with a healthful dose of serotonin in our brain). We often trust or feel safest around those who do not trigger our unconscious stress response—or as we're taught at a very young age, "stranger danger." We unconsciously respond to cues that indicate who is safe and who is not, based on how they look, talk, or behave, who tend to share and support our thoughts, feelings, and beliefs.

Just the same, we also avoid or reject those who don't make us feel safe, supported, or protected, who disagree with our thoughts, feelings, and beliefs, as subtle cues might indicate, by the way they look, talk, or behave.

This unconscious response happens instantaneously in every human being. We tend to consider someone who trusts and likes everyone as innocent or naïve, and consider someone who doesn't like or trust anyone as hateful, jaded, or bitter, with most people falling somewhere in between (depending on life experience and neurological development).

When there is a perceived threat, the amygdala gets signaled first, releasing stress hormones and neurochemicals like cortisol and adrenaline that prepare the body to fight or run away. At the same time, the activation of your amygdala also impairs the prefrontal cortex that is responsible for higher executive functioning, like emotional regulation, impulse control, critical thinking, and empathy. This is why when you feel threatened, scared, or angry, your heart races, your mouth feels dry, your muscles tense, and you might even jump or scream before you know what happened.

What often makes stressful influences extra difficult is the judgment of "good vs. evil"—that is, we tend to perceive harm done to someone who is "good" (or undeserving of harm) as an act of evil, while harm done to someone who is perceived as "evil" (or deserving of harm) as an act of good. We have empathy and understanding for the good (who does not trigger our unconscious stress response), but not for the evil (who does trigger our unconscious stress response).

Because of how the brain works, it is extremely difficult to empathize with someone who has caused us harm, and we have an unconscious survival instinct to stick with those who make us feel safe, to defend ourselves against those who pose a threat—reinforcing the "us" (good) vs. "them" (evil) paradigm.

This is also why it becomes extra complicated and confusing when hurt people hurt people—when those who've been hurt feel justified in hurting others.

When we don't allow ourselves to feel empathy for those who hurt us—that is, having an unbiased sense and understanding of the experience and condition of another—we inhibit our own ability to understand, heal, and prevent further harm.

It's not just a matter of willpower.

Even though we have the most access to information than any

other time in human history, we also have access to the most divisive, angry, scary, challenging, abusive, traumatic, and threatening information than any other time in history as well.

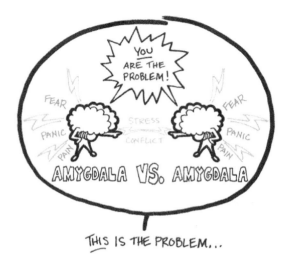

THIS IS THE PROBLEM...

When our attention is pulled and stretched in so many different ways (especially digitally), we become more stressed and less tolerant of people who trigger our unconscious stress response. We become increasingly impatient due to our increased need for immediate reward to reduce our stress response. It's a bit of a self-sustaining cycle of problems, when the source of our stress (whether our computer, phone, job, coworkers, community, home, or family) is also the source of our safety, security, and reward.

What we haven't yet developed are healthful ways to moderate consumption of such massive amounts of information, to healthfully navigate all of the stress-inducing influences that come our way, in every form, from every direction—including socially, environmentally, nutritionally, and chemically (S.E.N.C.).

This is the focus of mental fitness.

The "us vs. them" paradigm relates directly to how competing parts of your brain operate, namely the amygdala versus the prefrontal cortex. As previously discussed, your amygdala and prefrontal cortex are two of the most important parts of your brain to understand when it comes to developing healthful thoughts, feelings, and behaviors.

When left unrecognized and untreated, chronic stressors can lead to more serious mental and behavioral health conditions. Acts of violence and aggression are often related to emotional pain, trauma, bullying, and ridicule, and a need for power and control to mitigate the unconscious stress response by fighting rather than fleeing. While violent or aggressive behaviors are not mental illnesses in themselves, they may be related to a deeper brain health condition that poses serious risks to one's mental health.

Does this mean that EVERY person who is traumatized, bullied, or ridiculed will develop a serious mental health condition? No.

Does this mean that EVERY person who struggles with a mental health condition will develop a mental illness or become violent? Nope.

Our genetics and life experiences are as diverse as the people we are, that impact our physiological and neurological health and development in different ways.

That's also why understanding mental health as an aspect of brain health is so important. When we don't provide proper care and healing neurologically and physiologically, we increase the risk of more serious mental and behavioral health conditions, including harm toward self and others.

There are many ways to mitigate the impact of stressors on the brain, that can impact mental and behavioral health, including self-awareness, seeking safety and social support, prioritizing rest and nourishment, and of course, accessing mental health care and therapy to support healing and resilience.

Without awareness or access to these critical health services and practices, the impact of emotional trauma will continue to manifest in unhealthy ways, including violent behaviors.

The topic of violence and mental health can be extremely uncomfortable and mentally challenging due to the stress response involved, especially if you are the victim or target of violence.

What's often lacking in conversations about violence and mental health, which could help reduce this stress response, is awareness of brain health, function, healing, and well-being, and why we think, feel, and behave the way we do.

If you find this topic challenging or uncomfortable, please know that is normal. Your brain is working hard to understand thoughts and feelings of someone who poses a perceived threat to you, making it difficult for your prefrontal cortex to consciously process.

Mental fitness practices are critical in promoting both brain health and mental well-being.

It's important to remember that mental health is as much about brain health as it is behavioral health and healing, whether from emotional trauma, chemical imbalance, or any number of other psychological, physiological, or neurological conditions, that can affect neurological or physiological activity, including perceptions, thought patterns, attitudes, and behaviors.

Just as we must understand the root causes of cancer and car accidents to save lives, so must we understand the root causes of violent behaviors to provide proactive care, treatment, and prevention to save lives.

We must continue to have uncomfortable conversations to exercise and develop our brains in healthful ways, just as we would a muscle—to share more, learn more, and know more—because knowledge is both powerful and healing, when practiced and applied in healthful ways.

While the process of adaptation involves responding to stress by developing healthful coping skills (i.e., thoughts, feelings, habits, and behaviors) to navigate changes in our lives in healthful ways, conformity is when we demand that others think, feel, look, act, or otherwise be like us in order to be accepted as part of a group—to maintain the group's power, influence, and control. Conformity is the result of stressors that trigger the unconscious "fight, flight, or freeze" response in the amygdala, that emotionally manipulate you to surrender for our own safety and protection. Threats or intimidation might be used to force or pressure people into repressing their own personal power, thoughts, and feelings, in order to be accepted or protected by the group.

If history has taught us anything, it's that forcing people to conform by emotionally manipulating their thoughts, feelings, beliefs, and behaviors via their stress response—without consideration of the long-term impact on their health and well-being (physically and mentally)— causes long-term harm and long-lasting damage.

Being forced to change and give up one's personal power and autonomy to another, in order to survive without adequate time to adapt and prepare, without healthful reward and reinforcement, without any long-term health benefits, can be detrimental to one's health, success, and well-being—not to mention the health, success, and well-being of the greater community that is forced to conform.

The reward must also be healthful and intrinsic in value to reinforce long-term healthful habits, attitudes, and behaviors.

Thriving takes effort and practice, to feel and do one's best in their environment, within their abilities and what they have. In essence, to thrive is to adapt, and to adapt is to thrive. If one is not thriving, then one is not adapting.

Adaptation is not as simple as saying, "Get over it," or, "Embrace change."

Adaptation is a challenging neurological and physiological process, but we are also wired for it, otherwise known as neuroplasticity (that is, the way neurons can adapt to fire in more healthful ways to achieve desired health outcomes). Your body and brain just need time, with experience, exposure, repetition, reward, and reinforcement—that are the building blocks of developing any new healthy habit.

The difference between surviving and thriving might seem small, but it's actually rather large.

Right now, somewhere out there, someone is fighting cancer. They may have lost their hair from the effects of chemotherapy, and they may have received a scary prognosis, but they are determined to not let fear get the best of them.

They are not just surviving but thriving, by making the most of each day with every healthful step they can take. They are receiving medical treatments and educating themselves in ways to support their healing and recovery, including exercising when they feel well enough to do so. They are finding ways to reduce stress as best they can and finding ways to stay optimistic by avoiding pessimism and unhealthy influence. They are spending time with people they love and laughing at the funny things in life. They are balancing their body chemistry to support their immune system, increasing their ability to heal and fight disease that improves their odds of recovery. There is no guarantee how much time they have, but they are making the most of the time they do have, which is what thriving is all about.

At the same time, somewhere out there, a physically fit athlete is struggling emotionally, with anxiety and depression, an eating disorder, steroid abuse, and body dysmorphia, with a failing marriage and thoughts of suicide, too afraid to tell anyone or reach out for help. Every day is a battle to survive, even though they appear to be physically fine.

This comparison is not about right versus wrong, or better or worse.

This comparison is an example of how often we misinterpret and misunderstand the concept of fitness, by only focusing on the physical, that can be a detriment to our health, healing, and well-being. Our society is obsessed with physical appearance, and we punish "bad" behaviors without understanding the brain health or function behind it.

Without proper understanding and care for the brain, we struggle to survive, much less thrive.

When we learn about human history, it comes as no surprise why a free society is so challenging and uncomfortable, and why we so often take it for granted and forget that, thinking that something is wrong when it becomes challenging and uncomfortable, and we jump right back into old patterns of trying to get rid of those who challenge us and make us uncomfortable.

No matter how moral, just, or righteous we think we are, every human brain has an amygdala that triggers an unconscious stress response, and every human brain has a prefrontal cortex that becomes impaired (more or less) when we don't manage our stress response in a healthful way. We all must be aware of our own unconscious stress response to set a healthful example and teach others how to navigate stress, challenges, and discomfort in healthful ways.

It is so much easier for our human brains to believe we are always right and justified, and always an exception to any rule, while others are not—how "they" are always guilty and "we" are always innocent.

This is why it is very difficult and stressful for the human brain to admit fault or wrong-doing when we are in a stressed state, with inhibited empathy, comprehension, and compassion for the other person. We often fight each other, even to the death, when each believes that they are right and justified, and the other is guilty and to blame. When we don't take accountability for our own unconscious stress response, we can perceive anyone who tries to tell us otherwise as a threat, by challenging our brain. They instantly become our enemy, and someone to eliminate, attack, or avoid.

There's maybe no experience quite as universal or illustrative as our unconscious stress response while driving. You know, that feeling you get behind the wheel when driving at high speeds, and your conscious brain doesn't have to think much about operating the vehicle.

When driving, your conscious attention might be focused instead on things like whether you'll be early or late to your destination, or what you have to do when you get there. Maybe you're listening to the radio or singing along to a song. Maybe you're talking to whomever else is in the car, or thinking about a conversation or fight you just had with someone. Maybe you're talking on the phone or attempting to do a Google search while you drive.

We often describe driving on "autopilot" as a function of our unconscious nervous system—as a sort of muscle memory with those activities we do over and over again that require less and less conscious effort. Since our unconscious nervous system is also connected to our unconscious stress response, we are automatically in a defensive state while driving too, with our unconscious stress response ready to burst. You might feel a surge of anger when someone cuts you off, drives too close, or drives too fast or slow.

We don't consciously see the other cars as fellow humans, but as obstacles in our way. When we are operating on "autopilot" (via our autonomic nervous system), we automatically perceive every other vehicle as a threat or obstacle in our way, as barriers preventing us from getting where we want to go.

Maybe you've cursed, tailgated, or flipped off another driver out of anger while driving, only to realize later that it was your friend, coworker, or relative (sorry, Grandma!).

The reason that freedom requires continual conscious work and effort is because of the natural unconscious stress response of the human brain. Like every other animal in nature, humans will always get stressed when inhibited, limited, trapped, tired, hungry, cornered, attacked, threatened, or otherwise offended by those perceived as a threat, who do not think, feel, or behave the way we want them to, as part of the "us vs. them" paradigm, when we see other people are barriers and obstacles to our goals and desires.

Mental fitness is an essential part of success and well-being for every person, even those who don't think, feel, or behave like you, and maybe even get in our way.

Freedom means having the ability to fully "be" and embrace your honest authentic human self, even when others don't like you, or disagree. Freedom means being able to love and care for yourself completely—inside and out—to feel and do your best, even in the face of obstacles, challenges, and adversity. Freedom is the ability to express your thoughts and feelings openly and honestly—without fear of persecution. Freedom is the ability to disagree, even when it might create conflict (that can trigger an unconscious stress response too). Freedom is not being forced to conform under pressure or intimidation to think, feel, or behave as others do, in order to be accepted or protected by a particular person or group of people.

Freedom is the ability to do all of this, to navigate the ups and downs of life in healthful ways, even when we feel stressed.

The same unconscious stress response is what puts freedom in jeopardy too. When we feel and do better with less stress or challenge from others, it can seem like a quick and easy fix to just eliminate them.

As natural as it might be for our very human brains to desire dominance and superiority, in order to ensure our own safety and security to ease our unconscious stress response, limiting freedoms in the short-term also has long-term brain health implications by triggering an even greater unconscious stress response (as illustrated by human history).

Freeing yourself really requires freeing others as well, in order to ease the unconscious stress response in all.

This just might be the greatest human struggle. When we're not free to be who we are, we cannot feel and do our best, and we all suffer for it mentally, emotionally, socially, physically, and economically—because of how it impacts brain health and function.

That feeling of discomfort from your brain being challenged is the feeling of freedom, since freedom for you means freedom for others too, which is why a free civilized society is so challenging and uncomfortable to maintain, when trying to balance a sense of liberty and freedom with a sense of safety, justice, and civility—to minimize everyone's unconscious stress response and optimize everyone's prefrontal cortex.

So, the next time someone says or does something you don't like that triggers your unconscious stress response, STOP for a moment and breathe, to help calm your amygdala and engage your prefrontal cortex. Try to empathize with the feelings and experiences of others to comprehend the situation, while maintaining the safety and boundaries you need to think critically and understand why you feel the way you do too.

14 CULTURE AND CONNECTION

Would you rather spend time with people who agree or disagree with you? (Be honest.)

In other words, would you rather spend time with people who make you feel accepted or rejected?

As human animals, we tend to feel safest and most comfortable with those who embrace and accept us, who feel safe and familiar, due to how the human brain works. We tend to associate with those who seem to think, feel, and behave like us to avoid the threat of conflict, disagreement, and distress.

Unfortunately, this very natural tendency also perpetuates the stress and dissonance we feel with the unfamiliar, by preventing us from experiencing those new (and often uncomfortable) experiences that shape and influence our neurological perception, and allow us to adapt—to broaden our sense of who and what are safe and familiar. This is probably the greatest challenge of diversity and inclusion as well—when differences trigger stress, conflict, and disagreement, and ultimately lead to rejection, exclusion, and avoidance.

Rather than avoiding differences as an unconscious stress response, the healthful practice is to learn why we feel that way (without stress-inducing shame or judgment) and how to consciously navigate differences in more healthful ways, whether playing together, being creative together, or by sharing stories that foster a greater sense of understanding, familiarity, safety, connection, and empathy.

While our "winner-takes-all" culture might teach us that life is a competition that requires many to lose in order for one or a few to win, thriving in life actually requires collaboration. We often fail to realize that being a "loser" is actually a good and healthful thing when it's an indication of one's attempt, effort, and learning experience that will hopefully encourage them and not discourage them to try again—to learn, practice, and adapt each time, to improve their own performance, regardless of anyone else's.

If only it were that easy to change cultural norms, right?

When an influence is as systemic as culture, it's important to realize the power and influence you have, and what's also outside of your control (namely the weather and other people). Culture connects us emotionally with those who share it—past, present, and future—that becomes part of our self-perceived identity as well. Your thoughts, feelings, and behaviors are influenced by culture as much as your thoughts, feelings, and behaviors reinforce and influence that system—a cyclical relationship powered by each and every brain in the culture.

Culture is the combination of societal systems that influence populations of people far more than any one individual is able to influence or change. Culture may connect those who share the same systems of language, economics, currency, mathematics, government, leadership, religion, beliefs, goals, purpose, and traditions (to name a few). This is why culture change is so challenging, slow, and gradual, and requires the conscious effort of a social collective, often called a "movement."

When trying to change or challenge a culture, we are essentially attempting to change and challenge every human brain that is influenced by that system, including beliefs, traditions, and personal identity, that automatically triggers an unconscious stress response and neurological resistance. While we can witness and observe the physical manifestation of social conflict, we cannot easily witness or observe the neurological driver of the conflict in the brain without conscious effort, learning, comprehension, and understanding (that becomes more difficult when our unconscious stress response is triggered).

While we might embrace those who embrace our culture, we may feel threatened by those who reject it, who have a loyalty to their own, that is just as much part of their personal identity.

When cultural traditions and beliefs are figuratively and literally set in stone, separating "us" from "them," then it's incredibly difficult to create a culture of inclusion that unites rather divides, when cultural traditions and beliefs do not allow change or challenge—not just on one side, but all, as a collective.

A healthful social environment is critical to the health and development of every human brain, since a large part of our environment is other people. So we defend and protect what we feel is safe and healthful (that doesn't trigger our stress response).

Like everything that humans create, sometimes culture is healthful, and sometimes it's not. Therefore, cultures must be allowed to change and adapt as the people they influence do too, to maintain a healthful environment, as we continue to live, learn, and grow.

The greatest value and benefit of cultural tradition seems to be how it allows us to learn and appreciate where we came from, to learn from and appreciate humans who came before us, to appreciate all they endured without the information, resources, or experiences that we now have access to today, thanks to their hard work. As imperfect as modern life still might be (and always will be, since humans are complex creatures), appreciating our cultural heritage is a form of practicing gratitude. The fact that you're reading this book right now says a lot (for which I am grateful as well).

The tough questions remain … How do we change, create, or adapt a culture without sacrificing an old one, and losing our sense of identity, connection, heritage, and gratitude? If the point of culture is to maintain traditions and beliefs that are central to our identity, then how do we develop new ones without losing our heritage and history?

Without a "restart" or "refresh" button, how do we move forward into the future when we are so tied to our past? How do we avoid cultural conformity and appropriation to preserve what's healthful while getting rid of what's not? And who decides?

Do we really need to share the same language, dialect, race, gender, age, experiences, abilities, education, perspective, ideology, religion, beliefs, goals, styles, currency, class, or economic status to respect, embrace, and appreciate each other?

Whether or not other people think, feel, or believe the same as you, the most important part of the human experience is to stay curious, to activate your prefrontal cortex by asking, "Why?" as much as, "Why not?"

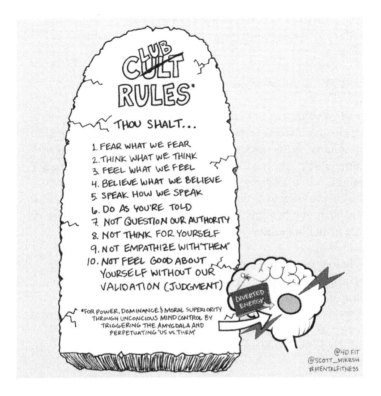

This is also an important self-defense practice to avoid the perils of social influencers, cults, and extremist groups that most notably discourage critical thinking, empathy, change, and challenge. Emotional awareness is critical to realizing, avoiding, and resisting emotional abuses, grooming, and manipulation that pose a real threat to your physical and mental health, safety, and well-being, especially when emotional tactics are so often slow, stealthy, seemingly innocent, and gradual—until they are not.

If the person or group you associate with uses emotional tactics to first allure you and then intimidate you into compliance, conformity, or agreement that makes you doubt or question your own judgment and critical thinking abilities—

this is a RED FLAG. If you are not allowed to doubt their authority or ask challenging questions, this is another RED FLAG.

And why is this all important to know?

It all goes back to understanding and navigating your unconscious stress response. When you practice emotional awareness, stress management, and stress reduction, you are better able to perceive yourself and others as fellow human beings, not just barriers or obstacles. When we engage the healthful abilities of our prefrontal cortex, we can create, learn, and share the benefits of cooperation to survive and thrive on this planet, together.

Whether our differences are based on experience, genetics, neurology, physiology, trauma, impairment, imbalance, or illness, they all require regulating the unconscious stress response of our amygdala to activate and engage our prefrontal cortex, to optimize comprehension, compassion, critical thinking, and problem solving—to promote health, safety, and well-being.

15 WHAT ABOUT SPIRITUALITY?

Scientifically speaking, nature is energy, and you are a natural energetic organism. That means energy is in and all around you, in one form or another, and influences your health and well-being every second of every day.

The energy that influences your thoughts, feelings, attitudes, and behaviors affects your health and environment in measurable ways. While healthful energy that you consume and transmit contributes to growth and well-being, any toxic energy that you consume or transmit also contributes to illness and destruction.

Spirituality can be a sensitive subject to discuss and analyze for many reasons. One of these reasons is because our sense of spirituality is often reinforced by deep emotions that provide a sense of trust, purpose, safety, comfort, and connection, that are reinforced and repeated throughout our lives. With emotions neurologically connected to our autonomic (or unconscious) nervous system, when our emotions are challenged or threatened, it can trigger an unconscious emotional stress response.

Since we often learn about spirituality and religion long before we learn about brain health and function, and our personal identity and purpose in life are so often connected to our spiritual beliefs and religious practices, discussing brain function can challenge those long-held beliefs that have also been neurologically repeated and emotionally (neurochemically) reinforced.

As human beings, we also have an innate stress response to death and the unknown, which is why topics that address life and death can be especially stress-inducing. Spirituality is one of those topics that can be deeply personal and diverse across different cultures, religions, traditions, and belief systems, with faith in a "higher power" than what science has yet to discover.

With so much about the human condition to still explore and discover, we still rely very much on faith as a form of trust. Faith isn't just limited to spirituality or religion. We can have faith in science, each other, and ourselves, or all of the above, including spirituality, God, and religion. What you personally have faith and trust in is as unique as you are.

Rather than challenging spiritual practices and beliefs, exploring and understanding brain health and function must really be considered a part of and not a replacement for spiritual practices, since science has proven time and again that the energy inside and around all of us is an essential part of human health, function, and well-being. Energy powers your brain and body from the food you eat to the water you drink, from the light waves you see to the sound waves you hear, from the air you breathe to the sunlight you absorb, and even the energy we feel and share with each other.

What can be unhealthful and damaging is when we use and justify practices that are mentally, emotionally, or physically abusive in the name of spiritual health and healing, whether through violence, alienation, or oppression in the name of righteousness—to save one's soul—without understanding or considering the complex neurological and physiological functions of one's brain and body.

Most devastating is when practices intended to heal the spirit lead to mental or physical pain, trauma, and even death.

That's not to say by any means that all spiritual practices or religious beliefs are unhealthy or harmful. Spiritual practices can, in fact, be quite healthful by promoting healthful thoughts, feelings, and behaviors, even when we don't know why (and still allowed to ask).

Most spiritual practices actually include stress-relieving mental fitness practices like practicing peace, love, hope, purpose, mindfulness, meditation, gratitude, forgiveness, emotional regulation, impulse control, compassion, acceptance, music, social support, and community connection—that all promote brain health and mental function by calming our unconscious stress response and sympathetic nervous system.

Discussing brain health and function in an inclusive and non-judgmental way is an important mental fitness practice in itself, regardless of one's spiritual beliefs. Whatever differences we might have in our beliefs, our brains still function in much the same way, with energy passing between our conscious and unconscious mind that influences how we think, feel, and behave.

Different spiritual beliefs, practices, and traditions that promote health, healing, and well-being are an important part of health, healing, and well-being for many people; maybe even for you.

To be truly inclusive, however, I want everyone who reads this book to feel understood and respected, including YOU—whether you identify with a specific faith, religion, spiritual practice, or not. I acknowledge and respect your beliefs, whatever they might be now or in the future, and leave the topic of spirituality totally up to you.

The mental fitness practices outlined in this book are designed to be as relevant, useful, and effective in promoting brain health and well-being whether you incorporate spirituality or not, based on what you need to help you feel and do your best, to achieve your goals, to live your life to the fullest, as a vital and valuable human being.

BALANCE

Level One: Balance

☐ **Feel your feelings to be emotionally aware**

☐ **Shed shame and stigma by facing your fears**

☐ **Move your body to rebalance your body chemistry**

☐ **Talk or journal to process thoughts and feelings**

Mental fitness practices are not about controlling your thoughts and feelings (or someone else's), but rather understanding what influences them so you can increase the healthful influences (that help you feel balanced) and minimize the unhealthful influences (that make you feel unbalanced).

Practicing mental balance is much like navigating a hot air balloon, with internal and external forces that you must be aware of to stay afloat and safely make your way through stressful pressure changes and turbulence.

Even the most experienced navigators can face challenges and accidents when the stress is stronger than anticipated. What's most important is your ability to stay afloat or land safely, to walk away and recover to get where you want to go.

Much like navigating a vehicle, it's important to know how your brain and body work together to optimize operations, including any neurological or physiological challenges, imbalances, or sensitivities you might have. These neurological and physiological responses are your body's way to regain balance and homeostasis, to get back to a more healthfully balanced state.

Being aware of the mental "weight" you are carrying and how

you perceive and process it can help you work toward a healthfully balanced neurological and physiological state that involves engaging your prefrontal cortex to regulate your stress response (by calming your amygdala). Identifying the source of your stress and pressure is the first step in knowing what's throwing you off-balance. Similar to physical balance, it's not always the amount of weight you carry but how you carry it that can cause imbalance.

It's important to be aware of the thoughts, feelings, and information you are processing to process and rebalance your neurology and physiology in a healthful way—to optimize and energize your prefrontal cortex. Overloading yourself with stress-inducing thoughts, feelings, and information that do not contribute to your health and well-being can have unhealthy consequences, unless you know how to navigate them in a healthy way to lighten the load.

While it's neither possible nor healthy to avoid every stress in life (since there are healthful forms of stress like excitement and anticipation, and your stress response is essential to avoiding threats to your health and well-being), it is critical to your health and well-being to be aware and learn how to cope, adapt, and minimize the impact of toxic stressors in your life—including your social, environmental, nutritional, and chemical influences (S.E.N.C.).

Anger, resentment, and hostility are examples of toxic emotions that can inhibit your health and healing, with elevated levels of cortisol, due to prolonged stress that contributes to a number of mental, physical, and neurological health conditions.

When practicing balance, try to recognize and reduce your sense of fear, worry, shame, guilt, envy, or blame that trigger the unconscious stress response of your amygdala. Being aware of how and why you feel the way you do is an important step in regulating your stress response to achieve a more healthful neurochemical balance.

16 EMOTIONAL AWARENESS

You feel emotions for a reason, and you can't always control your emotions for a reason.

Your unconscious emotions are meant to guide and protect you, but at times they may also consciously confuse and deceive you when you don't know how or why you feel the way you do.

Emotions are neither "good" nor "bad" in themselves since they are simply a natural neurochemical response to some neurological or physiological stimuli. While you may not be able to consciously control your unconsciously driven emotions, you can certainly learn to understand, manage, navigate, and express them in healthful ways to achieve healthful outcomes, to feel and do your best.

Your thoughts, feelings, and behaviors are a neurological response to your internal and external environments. By internal environment, I mean your body chemistry and neurological condition. How you interpret and act on your feelings is what determines whether you achieve a healthful outcome or not. Your external environment includes your physical and social environment, including the food, beverages, air, chemicals, sensory stimulation (such as light, sounds, smells, touch, and taste) and even information you consume.

When you make a decision based on how you feel about a particular person, thing, or situation, rather than impartial facts and information, it's considered a biased decision—driven by unconscious emotion.

When you are conscious and thoughtful about your behaviors, and you make decisions based on impartial facts and information (even when it challenges your thoughts and feelings about that person, thing, or situation), it's considered an unbiased decision—driven by critical thinking that is a function of your conscious mind (that may contradict your unconscious emotion).

Being aware of your amygdala and unconscious stress response is an important part of emotional awareness. Even more important is to be aware without triggering your own unconscious stress response with feelings of shame or judgment (since you're only human!).

Paying conscious attention to your emotions, without shame or judgment, allows you to discover why you feel the way you do by engaging your prefrontal cortex, even when your emotions seem confusing or irrational in the moment.

In order to find the solutions and answers you need, you first need to calm your amygdala to fully engage your prefrontal cortex. What often prevents us from acceptance and learning is fear and shame—by triggering the amygdala and impairing the prefrontal cortex.

We're often taught that "actions speak louder than words" because it's so easy to say one thing and do another, when it's really our behaviors that have the most physical impact. Right?

Since ninety percent of brain activity operates without conscious awareness, it's much easier for us to rationalize our behaviors AFTER they take place than it is to know how we'll behave in advance, when none of us really know how we'll feel in advance.

(That also contributes to anxiety.)

This can make our thoughts, feelings, and behaviors seem contradictory, hypocritical, or irrational to others.

For example, how often have you told others to be their authentic selves, to love themselves, and to not worry what others think, only to turn around and get mad at someone and call them names for disagreeing with you or not doing what you want them to do?

It's nothing to feel ashamed about, since we all have at some point in our life, but it is something that requires conscious awareness in order to manage your unconscious stress response in a more healthful way, to achieve healthful outcomes.

How many times do we say or hear, "Why did you do that when you said you wouldn't?!"

With the response being, "I don't know!"

Even finding the right words can be difficult when your head is spinning with a surge of neurochemicals and emotions.

In fact, there are no words in your brain until your conscious mind assigns those you've learned to your abstract thought or feeling, with the appropriate neurochemical signals (AMAZING, right?!).

This is why we cry and scream as babies when we have no words, or when our unconscious stress response as an adult feels too overwhelming to process.

We are not consciously aware of our unconscious feelings until we actually make an effort to be conscious of them, often after they've been expressed in our emotions and behaviors, that we may not consciously understand either.

Critical thinking is an important part of processing, which includes emotional awareness driven by the prefrontal cortex, that must be practiced, exercised, and developed like any other fitness level or life skill—including the ability to ask what, why, and how.

Maybe you caught yourself in the moment and managed to pause and process, maybe counted to ten, took a deep breath, focused your mind on the problem in front of you, and tried to navigate the stressful situation with your best intent, to avoid causing further harm or damage. This is why engaging your prefrontal cortex through emotional awareness, controlled breathing, and stress reduction techniques are so important to help calm, balance, and heal the neurochemical response throughout your body and your amygdala.

It's extremely unhealthy and unrealistic to expect humans to control their emotions just by wanting it, as though controlling our emotions is a sign of emotional strength—when it's often quite the opposite. When our fear-based unconscious stress response due to shame, stigma, and social expectation leads to repress thoughts and feelings rather than encouraging us to impress them in healthful ways, our health and well-being can suffer, including our mental, emotional, behavioral, and physical health.

Mindfulness is the practice of processing thoughts and feelings in a healthful way by engaging our prefrontal cortex.

Emotional awareness and emotional processing is a critical part of mental fitness, whether through talking or journaling on your own, with a friend, coach, or colleague, or with the help of a licensed therapist. It takes conscious effort and practice to notice your unconscious thoughts and feelings, to express and process them in healthful ways, to understand and regulate them, by engaging your prefrontal cortex to calm your unconscious stress response, to develop more healthful behaviors.

This is why being able and allowed to talk about your thoughts and feelings is a critical part of brain health and mental well-being—to achieve a healthier neurochemical balance or homeostasis.

An important practice for achieving mental balance is to recognize and acknowledge your emotions, even when you may not fully understand them. Imagine being lost at sea and suddenly seeing a boat on the horizon. You have a sudden sense of hope and relief that you'll be seen and saved. You're still floating at sea, but in that instant, your emotions change with a rush of neurochemicals that help calm your unconscious stress response.

We often have unconscious expectations without realizing the unconscious stress response that those expectations have on ourselves and others. For example, expecting something to be easy means your brain and body don't prepare for more than you can easily do without preparation, with little threat of failure to motivate you. You are therefore more likely to attempt something you perceive as easy since there is no perceived threat or risk of failure.

If your expectation is met, then your perception is reinforced. Since you had perceived the task to be easy, however, with a rather low neurochemical response to start, you may only feel a tiny bit of satisfaction. Due to this lower neurochemical response, you will also feel a lower sense of reward, and may not want to do it again.

On the other hand, if you fail at something you expect to be easy, your stress response might:

a) FIGHT, with an adrenaline rush that makes you feel more motivated and determined to prepare and try again, or...

b) FLEE, with cortisol inducing a sense of frustration and discouragement that prevents you from trying again.

For this reason, expecting something to be easy may increase the likelihood that you will try, but also increases the likelihood that you will lose motivation to try again if you fail.

On the other hand, when you expect something to be challenging, you may:

a) FIGHT, with an adrenaline rush that makes you feel motivated and determined to try your best, or...

b) FLEE, with cortisol inducing a sense of frustration and discouragement from even trying.

If you think you just read the same reactions twice, you did. That's the neurochemistry of your unconscious stress response that drives both the thrill of a challenge and the disappointment of defeat, or unmet expectations.

Similarly, it's often said that there is a thin line between love and hate—or in other words, between our prefrontal cortex and our amygdala. It's not so much a thin line as the relative change in our neurochemistry, resulting in a more or less severe increase or decrease in neurochemicals that can more or less trigger our unconscious stress response.

For example, when you feel safe and suddenly feel threatened, that's a more drastic neurochemical change than if you didn't feel safe to begin with, and you were on the lookout for a threat. Imagine a surprise party that you are not expecting, compared to a surprise party you are expecting, and how your stress response differs. It's not that you're more likely to hate those you love, but rather that those you love are more likely to cause a sense of deeper pain by the drastic change in our neurochemistry, because you didn't see it coming, and you no longer feel the sense of safety you once did.

The reason we can hurt the ones we love more easily is because the neurochemical impact of our behaviors on their emotions is more drastic as well. Consider the difference between a coworker getting mad at you compared to someone you love getting mad at you. You may feel more stress by the anger of your loved one, since the neurochemical change is much more dramatic when it starts at a higher level (like hitting a wall while driving 60 miles per hour, that causes severe damage and injury), compared to the neurochemical response triggered by your coworker (like hitting a wall driving 5 miles per hour, that's only a fender bender).

There is a saying that the difference between delight and disappointment is the difference between expectation and reality. When our expectations are met or even surpassed, we feel satisfied and delighted; and when our expectations are not met, we feel disappointed. Both are due to the relativity of neurochemical changes.

When someone we love and trust behaves in a way that does not meet our mental and emotional expectations, the change in our neurochemistry from high to low makes us feel more disappointed than those same behaviors would in someone we don't love or don't trust, since our neurochemical state was lower to start.

Likewise, when we have no expectation, we feel less

disappointed. Have you ever watched a movie you knew nothing about and enjoyed it more than a movie you had been excited to see after it had been hyped for months and months?

At the same time, we may also feel less motivated to try or make an effort, when we have low or no hope or expectation of success or reward. Then what's the point, right?

Does this all mean that we should set lower expectations for ourselves and others? Not necessarily. It all depends on the situation.

Setting challenging yet realistic expectations is an important mental fitness practice to maintain your sense of hope, reward, and motivation, since setting expectations that are unchallenging (too low) or unrealistic (too high) can have the opposite effect—by diminishing your sense of hope, reward, and motivation.

Finding the right balance is the key to maintaining a sense of hope, reward, and motivation that leads to success, based on every individual's personal needs, goals, desires, and abilities.

It's similar to the difference between someone laughing with you (as a sign of support) or laughing at you (as a sign of shame and offense). Humor and laughter can be either healthful or hurtful, depending on who is delivering and receiving it, and why. It all depends on the neurochemical response involved.

When laughter is perceived as a threat or act of mockery, then it triggers the unconscious stress response of your amygdala, that releases cortisol and adrenaline into your system and inhibits the higher functions of your prefrontal cortex. This is often associated with gaslighting, which is a form of emotional abuse.

Laughter perceived as a form of emotional support, on the other hand, helps relieve stress by stimulating the release of serotonin and dopamine that help calm your amygdala and energize the higher functions of your prefrontal cortex. While comedy "roasts" may seem harsh and cruel to the casual observer, those intimately involved who are "in" on the joke perceive it as a form of emotional support and stress relief, with those who love them making jokes about them to help lighten the mood and make other people who love them laugh. This is why humor and laughter must be practiced wisely, and why it's so important to know your audience—to know the difference between cruelty and comedy.

Smiling is a great way to stimulate a sense of contentment in yourself and others too, since our brains respond to the muscle movements in our face as a signal of happiness, safety, and contentment. We often feel a sense of happiness, safety, and contentment when someone smiles at us, that helps boost the release of serotonin and dopamine that lowers our unconscious stress response as well.

That said, when we are in a stressed state—maybe feeling forced to smile or feeling threatened by a particular person or group of people—smiling may trigger an unconscious stress response as a perceived threat in our attempt to keep our distance and defenses up, ready to fight or flee.

Telling someone who doesn't feel like smiling to smile is about as effective as telling someone who is in a stressed state to, "Just calm down." Unless you can lower their stress response with signs of empathy, compassion, and understanding, you will likely further trigger their unconscious stress response.

Emotional awareness isn't just about being aware of your own emotions, but the emotions of others as well, that is a cornerstone of emotional intelligence.

In my experience, smiling at someone in an attempt to share a sense of happiness, safety, and contentment can have a disappointing effect when they don't smile in return—when I expect them to smile back but they don't.

Rather than getting upset, the practice I use is to be consciously aware that in that moment, they may feel an unconscious stress response for a number of reasons, maybe because of how they perceive me, or from how they already felt from a previous stress-inducing experience. Maybe they just got fired, lost a loved one, had an accident, or had an argument with someone. They may not consciously intend to scowl at you and trigger your stress response, but that's just how they feel in that moment. Maybe they had a stressful day and just don't feel like smiling, or maybe they are neurologically different and don't perceive my smile as a sign of safety and comfort. Maybe they aren't even aware that I will perceive their scowl as a sign of apathy or aggression.

This is often what's meant by "don't take things personally" (that can trigger an unconscious stress response when we perceive it as an insult too).

A part of emotional intelligence is the ability to realize when someone else's thoughts, feelings, and behaviors have nothing to do with you personally, and everything to do with them, and what's going on inside of them. Even when someone says or does something that hurts you personally, the driver of their thoughts, feelings, and behaviors is not you but their brain that may be dealing with trauma, pain, imbalance, illness, or impairment.

The mental fitness practice of emotional awareness involves being consciously aware of your own feelings first, so you can reduce your stress response, and increase your ability to comprehend, think critically, and empathize with others. How others respond to you really has less to do with you as a person, and everything to do with how their brain is functioning and processing what they feel and perceive in that moment.

The most important part in the process of balance is learning as you go, from every success and failure, to develop your abilities and understand your limits. It's important to challenge yourself without risking your health or well-being, or the health and well-being of others. Practicing balance means getting back up when you fall, to try your best, to not get distracted by comparing yourself to others. Balance is all about navigating your own emotions, environment, and relationships, to feel and do your best, to achieve your own goals.

17 SHED SHAME AND STIGMA

When it comes to maintaining your well-being, shedding shame and stigma is a MAJOR mental fitness practice to promote brain health and neurochemical balance, with a sense of self-love, self-care, and self-acceptance. There are a whole lot of theories and beliefs about mental health and function that have contributed to a lot of fear, shame, blame, and confusion—that together have created a whole lot of stigma.

Shedding the shame you feel about yourself (or others) requires conscious effort to help reduce your unconscious stress response. By engaging your prefrontal cortex with various mental fitness practices, you can reduce the toxic level of cortisol in your system and increase healthful and healing neurochemicals like serotonin and dopamine.

When it comes to discussing the mind, shame and stigma often get in the way with value judgments that trigger our unconscious stress response. As previously mentioned, stress that triggers the amygdala can impair functions of the prefrontal cortex like empathy, creativity, comprehension, problem solving, emotional regulation, and impulse control, along with other cognitive, social, and metabolic functions—

especially for those already living with a mental health condition or brain disorder.

How the brain and body process thoughts, feelings, and nutrients has a direct impact on attitudes and behaviors—that directly impact wellness and inclusion, since response and outcomes can be different for different people.

Similarly, how different people feel and process shame can be different as well. In general, shame is a toxic, limiting, and counterproductive emotional response. Learning how to shed shame is an important part of promoting neurological balance, growth, and healing.

Shame is a tricky thing. It's essentially an act or sense of social aggression and punishment. Shame uses intimidation to trigger our unconscious stress response, in order to influence our thoughts, feelings, and behaviors out of fear—to comply, conform, or otherwise change our thoughts, feelings, and behaviors to those deemed moral or acceptable by those who shame us.

The main dysfunction of shame is the lack of healthful reward and reinforcement, and the harmful effect it can have on the unconscious stress response of the person being shamed.

Can you remember the last time someone shamed you? Did you do or say something "wrong" that others wanted you to change or stop? How did you feel? Did you stop? Did you change? Or did you just try to avoid that person or situation to not get caught?

Rather than reinforcing a desired behavior with a neurological reward, shame punishes an undesirable behavior, thereby triggering an unconscious stress response as a perceived threat and something we want to avoid. So while at first it might seem that shame helps prevent an undesirable attitude or behavior from happening again, it actually does nothing to neurologically reward, reinforce, or develop the desired healthful attitude or behavior, with the only reward being the avoidance of punishment.

For this reason, shame is deceptively counterproductive, since it rewards and reinforces avoidance rather than acceptance.

When the goal is to reinforce a more healthful attitude or behavior, shame is not the neurological solution.

When it comes to promoting healthier or more constructive attitudes and behaviors, reward, repetition and reinforcement are all needed to make us want to repeat that neurological experience until it becomes a habit.

Context and trust are everything. When we trust that someone has our best interest in mind, and wants us to succeed and be happy, we're less likely to take offense to otherwise shameful thoughts or comments. They might still sting, but you'll likely feel less defensive if you share a mutual respect and trust.

Different neurochemicals are released when the source isn't a perceived threat. We therefore often say more critical things to close family and friends (in the name of trust and honesty) than we would otherwise say to strangers, with whom we have not developed a sense of safety or trust. When we don't have a sense of mutual love, trust, respect, or safety with someone, we are more likely to perceive their criticism as a threat, triggering our unconscious stress response.

One practice to help reduce a sense of shame and offer more of a reward for success when offering advice is to use the phrase "would" (implying a choice as a recommendation) rather than the word "should" (implying an expectation or obligation).

The word "should" often packs an unintended connotation of guilt and shame, even when the intention is to provide guidance and encouragement.

For example, saying, "You should call them," implies that calling is an expectation or obligation for which you may be judged if you don't (tisk tisk), or that the person may be emotionally hurt or disappointed if you don't (double tisk).

On the other hand, "It would be good to call them," still has a sense of direction and urgency, but has a much lighter connotation as a choice for you to make. Part of this is because the person saying it is focusing on the act of calling rather than focusing on "you." Calling them would be a good thing to do, but there's no expectation or obligation to be judged. If you do call, you'll feel you did a good thing. If you don't call, there's no unmet expectation or sense of failure to feel ashamed about.

Dang, words are tricky when we can't see into the brains of the people sending and receiving. We so often forget that words can have different meanings to different people at different times in different situations. This variability of the unknowns is often what gets in the way of what we're trying to say. It might actually trigger our unconscious stress response as we struggle and stumble to find the right words when our amygdala gets in the way of our prefrontal cortex.

Speaking is different than communicating. Communicating can take many forms, with many layers, to effectively transfer knowledge from one brain to another. Like uploading and downloading data, a connection must first be made, so find those with whom you can connect.

Finding the right words can also be difficult under pressure, and may even trigger others who are trying to heal at the same time. When your brain is in a stressed state, words can feel like emotional landmines. When you're in a stressed state, you might unconsciously anticipate a threat and try to find one in self-defense. This unconscious effort to find something that validates your unconscious stress response is another form of confirmation bias.

For example, if someone told you, "You look nice today!" you could take it one of two ways—that you look particularly nice today, or that you haven't looked nice any other day. The implied meaning (or connotation) of the exact same words can change depending on the person, context, situation, intent, and implication, either perceived as a compliment or an insult.

Ultimately, the impact of the statement is in how the receiver perceives it, which may not be how the sender intended. If you're in a particularly good mood and having a particularly good day, your prefrontal cortex may be powerful enough to see the positive in the comment and take it as a compliment. If you're in a particularly bad mood and having a particularly bad day, your prefrontal cortex may be inhibited with your amygdala already fully charged and activated, and you are more likely to respond to the comment as a perceived threat and insult.

Another consideration for how we interpret words and emotions is the relationship between shame, guilt, and pity.

Do you remember a time you felt pity for someone, or someone expressed pity for you? How did you feel?

In a healthful and helpful context, guilt and pity may lead to a healthful outcome, if they promote healing and prevent future pain and suffering. In an unhealthful context, they may reinforce a toxic sense of shame.

It's not always the words alone that hurt, but the tone and intention.

Pity might seem sweet and innocent enough but can pack a painful punch. Pity may even be used mistakenly in place of compassion. It sure sounds like compassion with the sense of shared sadness it implies, but pity tends to imply a hierarchy or heir of superiority. We might pity those who have less or struggle more than we do, that in turn reinforces our own privilege and sense of superiority.

A rich person might pity a poor person, or a poor person might pity a rich person, in either case reinforcing what they have in terms of wealth, physical ability, love, or happiness by comparison.

Pity is usually a matter of comparison. We pity those less fortunate.

Compassion, on the other hand, has less to do with having less, or being inferior to a superior, and has more to do with a shared feeling or experience. To have compassion for someone means you care about their feelings, and don't want to injure or offend.

A compassionate act might actually be to avoid pity, and instead share your concern and respect.

Replacing the sense of pity with a sense of respect is a great way to reduce a sense of guilt or shame and increase a sense of trust and respect.

When we talk about a "toxic" attitude or behavior, we're most often referring to an attitude or behavior that involves shame. Shame is a toxic stress response because it acts like a venom to make you feel sick when you experience it (from elevated levels of cortisol), that makes you perceive yourself as the threat—a kind of auto-immune response in a sense. That neurochemical feeling of shame can have long-term health consequences (i.e., hypertension, hormone imbalance, irregular metabolism, anxiety, depression, etc.) if you don't properly shed it from your system, that requires conscious effort, emotional processing, and neurological healing (that may even require clinical therapy).

Shame is related to feelings of guilt, regret, and remorse since they are also stress responses. Unlike the feeling of shame, however, feelings of guilt, regret, and remorse stem from a sense of compassion for yourself and others (powered by the prefrontal cortex) that helps you identify and rectify the harm you may have caused, to help you reduce pain and stress in yourself and others (that also involves forgiveness of self and others).

The toxic feeling of shame, however, lacks a sense of compassion and forgiveness that are essential in the neurological healing process, and is a form of emotional punishment often based on a value or moral judgment toward self or others.
Shame is that lingering sense of dread, hopelessness, and stress that makes you feel you are unworthy of love, compassion, hope, healing, and forgiveness.

We often express shame toward ourselves or others in abusive ways, such as name calling, isolating, degrading, humiliating, bullying, or another form of physical or emotional abuse.

Why is it important to understand the health consequences of shame?

What we often shame most are behaviors that are driven by mental and emotional processes in the brain that we cannot see. Since we cannot see what's driving the behavior, it's hard for us to consciously understand and process, especially when the behavior triggers our unconscious stress response that inhibits our empathy and comprehension.

The behavior might even be driven unconsciously, whether by stress, trauma, illness, impairment, imbalance, or other neurochemical influence.

The most damaging part of shame is that it doesn't just judge the behavior, but the person as a whole. Shame doesn't just judge unhealthy influences, but judges the person who is impacted by them (that is really a form of victim-blaming).

For example, while we might understand the mental, emotional, and behavioral health consequences of shaming someone for being physically different, injured, scarred, impaired, unstable, or ill, we often still shame people for being or behaving mentally different, injured, scarred, impaired, unstable, or ill.

Since we tend to ignore what we don't know or can't see, we tend to overlook the inner workings, brain functions, or emotional struggles of people who don't "look" different, injured, scarred, impaired, imbalanced, or ill, and therefore tend to judge resulting behaviors rather than trying to understand them.

Why do we do this?

When we are not taught the basics of practical brain health and function, or why it's important to know and understand, it can be very difficult to notice or understand the driver of thoughts, feelings, and behavior—being our hidden brain and our internal neurochemical activity.

In all of my academic and professional education, never were all of the pieces put together in this way, to apply what we know, scientifically, to real life.

While we've come a long way in understanding the consequences of body shaming, we still have a long way to go in understanding the consequences of brain shaming too.

To call every brain health or mental health condition an "illness" is to limit our understanding and care, by not acknowledging the multiple sources of the pain. This lack of awareness has created a toxic stigma around mental health that perpetuates the pain and prevents proper care and healing.

There is never just one influence or issue in your life that needs care, navigation, and healing—but often several, all at the same time—that can make life feel overwhelming when you feel life is caving in on all sides.

Our society has gone too long without understanding the importance of prioritizing mental health, and we're all suffering the consequences.

You are the center of your life, and the care and healing starts there. Before trying to care for and heal others, you must first care for and heal yourself—one step at a time. Learn from the past and keep moving forward. If you need to disconnect or take a break from those who hold you back or aren't supportive, do it. You can reconnect or reunite when you (and they) are in a healthier state, if you choose. This is not just for your own good, but also for theirs. By taking care of yourself, you'll be better able to care for others and be a healthful example for them too.

If we really knew and understood how the brain works, we wouldn't shame people for their ignorance. Unfortunately most of us don't, and we do.

We often shame people for what they don't know when it's something we do know, or we believe it's something they should know and believe, and we may even feel offended by their lack of knowledge in some way. The practice of shaming, however, rarely results in agreement or understanding, due to the unconscious stress and defense response that shame triggers in the amygdala.

So we should ask ourselves, would we rather have people hide that they don't know something or share that they don't know without shame, so their brain is prepared to learn without stress or defensiveness?

Does it help to pretend we know when we don't? To nod in agreement when we don't, rather than asking curious questions to clarify?

Is it really wise to hide, deny, and lie? To fake it until you make it? To appear wiser and more capable than you really are?

Would you rather open someone's mind by reducing stress in preparation to learn, or would you rather feel righteous in your rightness, and have them feel stressed, shamed, insecurity, close minded, and confused?

An "open" mind is really an active prefrontal cortex. I use the acronym O.P.E.N. that stands for: Oxygenate, Process, Exercise, and Nutrition. A brain that is in distress or duress is in a defensive (or "closed") state neurologically, and is therefore not in an optimal state for critical thinking, empathy, problem solving, or comprehension. This applies to every age and every person, with important considerations to be made regarding brain health, function, and development—that are also impaired by shame.

We may be able to train ourselves to calm our amygdala when we're stressed to better engage our prefrontal cortex—by remaining calm in a crisis, controlling your breath or counting to 10, or focusing on a solution instead of the problem.

Mental fitness involves both challenging and essential life skills that must be developed much like training your body to lift a heavy weight or run a long distance.

Developing these life skills requires conscious effort and continual practice, that may also be harder for some than others. This is why patience, practice, and understanding are key.

18 FACING FEARS

Fear and worry are normal, but don't have to get in the way of you feeling or doing your best, or saying and doing what you need to get where you want to go. Practicing mental balance is a way to help navigate your unconscious stress response that's triggered by fear.

A healthful aversion to threats and danger can help keep you safe and protect you from harm, but how you perceive threats and danger is also related to how you manage stress. When you are stressed—whether from a threat, failure, loss, excitement, or anticipation—your amygdala is triggered, taking energy away from your higher-functioning consciousness powered by your prefrontal cortex.

Have you ever practiced a speech or presentation over and over again, and after you present it publicly, you barely remember presenting it? This is because when your unconscious stress response takes over, it impairs the short-term working memory of your prefrontal cortex and basically operates unconsciously—like you're on autopilot. This is why practice and preparation are so important to navigating stressful situations, to work with your stress response rather than against it.

Fear is a natural unconscious neurological stress response. Therefore, the term "fearless" is really another misnomer, since everyone experiences fear to some degree, as part of human brain function. The basic premise of fearlessness is the ability to navigate your unconscious stress response that is triggered by fear, not the absence of fear itself.

Do you remember the last time you felt surprised or afraid? How did you feel emotionally, mentally, and physically? Did you jump or scream? Did your heart race? Did you breathe faster (or even hyperventilate)? Did you start to sweat? Did you feel a sudden rush of energy or maybe even a little shaky or "out of control"? All of those things can happen when your unconscious sympathetic nervous system kicks in.

Was it easy for you to comprehend the situation, or did it take you a moment to collect your thoughts? If so, that's because comprehension is a power of your prefrontal cortex that also becomes inhibited when your sympathetic nervous system kicks in (triggered by your amygdala).

What did you do to regulate your emotions to navigate the situation safely and effectively? Maybe you closed your eyes or took deep breaths, which are two important practices to help rebalance your neurological system.

Whether or not you even knew it, you were practicing mental fitness!

Facing fears involves managing your stress response, which requires practice. It's not always easy, and you may not always have access to the tools or resources you need to safely reduce or eliminate the threat, but the driver to finding what you need is inside of you—your brain—including all of those neurochemicals that influence your critical thinking, problem solving, and motivation.

Your amygdala is triggered by stress signals before your conscious mind is aware of it, which is why you might scream or jump when you get frightened or scared. You might frantically look around to see what it was that scared you before you can calm down, and you feel a sense of relief and safety when you finally see it was just your friend playing a prank (at which time your unconscious stress response may include calling them a jerk).

Your brain and body have a way of storing long-term information about what harmed or threatened you to prevent it from happening again. It's a natural defense that is part of your neurology.

Your brain can be very selective in the information remembered and forgotten as well, depending on which part of the brain is activated. Long-term memory is connected to your unconscious stress response, and short-term working memory is connected to our conscious higher-functioning mind. This is why it's easier to remember a traumatic event than an everyday occurrence, and why we have to repeat lists of items we're trying to consciously memorize over and over again. With repetition comes reinforcement of those neuropathways that help convert short-term memory into long-term memory.

This is something we need to accept and embrace about ourselves and each other, as a part of human nature. We can't always control our memories or the emotional storms and turbulence we experience, but we can learn to navigate them better when we understand ourselves and each other better, for smoother sailing.

It's important to remember that you are organic and electrochemical, and constantly changing, just like the weather and every other part of nature. Even when you're not consciously aware, your brain and body are still moving, changing, growing, developing, healing, and adapting from countless internal and external influences.

The real danger is that when you are immersed in it and become acclimated to it, you may no longer notice the toxic harm being done that you need to get away from, like anything else that is toxic. You will continue to be exposed to the toxicity until you get out of that environment and allow your senses to readjust and acclimate to a more healthful environment.

Have you noticed how your body adapts to a cool pool? After you've been in the water for a while, the water suddenly feels so much warmer, and the air feels so much colder (as you rush for your warm towel!). Even better, have you ever jumped from a hot tub into a cool pool? Or jumped from a cool pool into a hot tub? The water feels hotter or colder depending on which your body acclimated to first, the cool pool or the hot tub.

Your brain and body unconsciously acclimate (or temporarily adapt) to your environment in much the same way, without you even knowing it. When things change, we feel differently, and the unconscious adaptation process begins.

This process can work for or against you—in healthful or unhealthful ways—depending on the nature and severity of the change. For example, if there's a toxic gas in the air, then it would be best to smell it to be aware of it, to get away from it. When you acclimate to the smell, however, and no longer notice it, then your health is actually at greater risk. It's the same when you're in an abusive relationship that becomes normalized after repeated exposure and abuse, and you no longer notice it, putting your health at greater risk too.

Similarly, when you are not able or allowed to consciously

notice and regulate your emotions by engaging your prefrontal cortex—through various means of emotional processing and self-expression—you may not notice when you "vent" or "explode" your unconscious emotions onto others. This is what contributes to a "toxic" environment, when our stress-induced emotions are thrown around like toxic litter, thereby triggering the unconscious stress response of others that may reinforce or soothe our stress response with a jolt of dopamine, as a sense of power and validation.

It's important to remember that while reducing the toxic impact of stress is critical to your health and well-being, stress itself isn't always bad, and can actually be a healthful motivator when your unconscious stress response kicks in to achieve a goal or seek help or safety. That rush of cortisol and adrenaline can be a very powerful motivator when it gets your brain and body ready for action, but it's also important to understand the effects of different stressors on your system.

Much like what you eat and drink, the effects of different kinds of stress can affect different people differently, which is why it's important to be aware of how different stressors affect you too. Some people might naturally have a higher neurological tolerance or adaptability for certain types of stressors that may affect other people differently. This is, in part, why some people might enjoy action-thrillers while others might find them unnerving (quite literally) and prefer comedies or less stressful entertainment instead.

You might also train your brain with various mental fitness practices to manage different kinds of stress more healthfully, thereby allowing you to process stress in more healthful ways than someone who has not trained or may have a different neurological disposition.

This is even more important in this information age, since the most damaging weapons of mass destruction aren't physical or chemical but psychological, in the form of disinformation and propaganda that can be instantaneously launched and consumed online, through various media, attacking and infecting millions of people all at once (arguably even more "infectious" than COVID-19 by the rate at which it can instantaneously be shared and spread).

Your power is your ability to influence, including your ability to question, verify, and validate what you've been taught and told, or how to think and feel, without shame or fear. Your power is your ability to process what you consume in healthful ways that allows you to cultivate a healthful life, by prioritizing your own health and well-being, and influencing others to do the same.

We have so much untapped brain potential, often because we are bombarded by stressful information that overloads our neurological system and impairs optimal brain performance, emotional regulation, and conscious mental function.

You might engage your prefrontal cortex by consciously closing your eyes for a moment and trying to breathe more slowly to calm yourself (and then kindly tell your friend to not scare you like that again). By consciously regulating your breathing, you are, in turn, calming your sympathetic nervous system to reengage your parasympathetic nervous system, to return your neurological activity to a more relaxed state, to activate your prefrontal cortex.

It's important to focus on mental fitness practices like mindfulness, emotional awareness, and controlled breathing to help navigate your unconscious stress response to engage your prefrontal cortex and conscious awareness, to be aware of those feelings, signals, and sensations that operate unconsciously beneath the surface and behind the scenes in your brain and body.

19 MOVE YOUR AMAZING BODY

Your brain and body are essentially one-in-the-same since your brain is part of your body, and one can't function without the other. Physical movement is as important for mental health and mental fitness as it is physical health and physical fitness, since it all relies on healthful neurological and physiological activity.

In fact, neurologically and physiologically speaking, the first fitness practice of any physical fitness program is actually a mental one, even when we may not realize it or define it as such. Since your brain is what drives your thoughts, feelings, and behaviors, healthful physical movement first requires healthful mental preparation, nourishment, rest, communication, planning, learning, confidence, accountability, encouragement, reward, and reinforcement—which is why we often rely on the emotional support and mental instruction of a fitness instructor, trainer, or coach.

We often say we need a personal trainer to help "whip us into shape" (that usually doesn't involve a physical whip, but a mental one).

Your thoughts and feelings are a vital part of developing healthful habits and behaviors, including healthful choices and movement. Repetition and reinforcement are ultimately what neurologically forge your thought patterns, expectations, habits, and behaviors, and being consciously aware of this is an important part of mental fitness.

When you realize how good you feel after walking, dancing, running, working out, or even just sitting up straight, those neuropathways are reinforced by a drip of feel-good neurochemicals, making you more likely to feel motivated to repeat it, as those neuropathways flow more easily with routine use and less resistance.

Since your brain and body are always working to achieve homeostasis and adapt to your environment, the more you exercise your heart, lungs, and muscles (that includes nourishment, rest, and recovery to promote growth and development) the stronger and more efficient they become, which goes for your brain as well. By increasing your heart rate and respiration, you increase blood flow to your brain and body that oxygenates and detoxifies your entire system, helping rebalance and release hormones and neurochemicals that help improve both mental and physical health and function.

Another important factor is that not only does your brain influence your body functions, but your body functions also influence your brain, unconsciously. Your heart and gut specifically have many neurological connections between them, which is why heart health and gut health are so connected to mental health. Eating well and reducing stress are two practices that are not only important for maintaining your physical health but also your brain health and mental function. (This is also why we say "follow your heart" and "trust your gut," since those powerful unconscious neurological connections send signals to your brain before you're even consciously aware.)

How you move or hold your body can be unconsciously influenced by your emotions just as your unconscious emotions can be influenced by your physical movement or posture, since your brain unconsciously responds to the position, function, and movement of your body.

For example, when you smile in a sincere way, your brain responds with a drip of dopamine that helps reduce stress and reinforces a feeling of contentment. This goes for whether the smile was in response to someone else smiling at you or if you are smiling as an exercise to reduce stress in yourself. That healthful release of neurochemicals helps reduce stress neurologically either way—whether your brain is responding to your facial muscles or your facial muscles are responding to your brain.

So the next time you feel bored, unmotivated, or insecure (even if that moment is right now), try the simple practice of sitting up straight with the best posture you can, to healthfully align your anatomy and neurological system, and see how your brain responds. Do you notice a subtle difference in how your brain and body feel? Do you feel a bit better emotionally too?

Whether the difference is 100% or 10%, any improvement is significant. Since the term "better" is always relative, what might be "better" for one person is always different than what is "better" for another. This is another reason why comparison is the thief of happiness and success. Above all else, please remember this when it comes to assessing your own happiness, success, and well-being. Your success is based on your own journey and rate of progress, no one else's.

20 USE WORDS AS TOOLS

What do you believe is the most powerful human invention ever created?

In my opinion, it's language—both written and spoken.

One of the most powerful abilities you have, unlike any other animal, is your ability to influence the thoughts, feelings, and behaviors of others by sharing your own thoughts and feelings, as well as learning from the thoughts and feelings of others through the power of language.

Words are critically important—even more than sticks and stones, since words can be used as tools or weapon as well, to hurt or heal. Contrary to that old nursery rhyme, words actually do cause neurological pain, trauma, and distress.

Whether we call it fighting, gaslighting, bullying, or abuse, words used as weapons can cause both short-term and long-term mental and emotional harm—neurologically and physiologically. The unconscious stress response in your brain can leave lasting mental and emotional scars neurologically, like an electrochemical burn that gets embedded deep into your long-term memory as part of your sympathetic nervous system.

While we might think language should be simple, perfect, and universal, it is not. Language is a tricky bugger in its imperfection.

Have you ever struggled to find the right words? Or have you said something that was not interpreted the way you intended?

There are essentially four parts to effective communication:

1) what you want to communicate
2) how you communicate it
3) how it's interpreted by the recipient
4) how the recipient responds (that then goes back to number one)

Communication is never a one-way street, and disruptions can occur at any point as it travels—whether on the sending or receiving end, or both.

What makes language even trickier is how we communicate in different ways with different people, depending on when, where, and how we learn, and how each brain in the communications matrix processes thoughts, feelings, and information in different ways—that can be as diverse and imperfect as the diverse and imperfect people we are.

Have you ever communicated with someone who spoke a different language? Or have you communicated with someone who processed thoughts and feelings differently, or struggled to communicate? Have you ever told someone you love that you hate them? Has someone ever said something to you in anger that they said they didn't mean the moment it came out (or after they calmed down)?

Emotional intelligence is especially critical in communications, to understand all of the human variables and influences involved, including the abstract emotions and sensory information behind it all, beyond simply the words being said, that may be limited in many ways.

The scientific term for modern-day humans is "Homosapien" that literally translated from Latin means "wise human."

So what makes you wise? And what does wisdom mean to you?

Wisdom is based on knowledge that comes from lived experience, critical thinking, and comprehension—all functions of your prefrontal cortex. It's not just the knowledge that makes you wise, however, but applying what you learn to your own life, to forge neuropathways in your brain that help you achieve healthful outcomes (the practice of good judgment).

Wisdom isn't simply copying or repeating "wise words" from a book, website, or lecture, but requires actually applying that information to your own life, to develop healthful judgment, habits, and behaviors. A wise person is one who practices what they preach or teach, which is also why it's hard to believe "words of wisdom" from someone who doesn't, and we tend to perceive them as dishonest or distrustful. For example, while you might know that eating fruits and vegetables is important to your health and well-being, unless you actually eat fruits and vegetables yourself, others will not perceive you as wise or trustworthy. Distrust triggers an unconscious stress response that inhibits your ability to comprehend and empathize, which makes learning from another's experience that much harder.

Similarly, someone who uses their freedom in ways that result in unhealthy outcomes is not considered wise by standard definitions of the word. Poor or unhealthy judgment is not wise at all, but rather unwise.

What makes you wise is your capacity to learn and apply what you learn to behave, create, communicate, and adapt in healthful ways to achieve healthful goals. Your wisdom has tremendous power and influence among those who trust you as well.

Early humans created advanced forms of verbal and written language, not only to alert and inform others in our tribe, but to pass on lessons learned from their own life experience, from one trusted person or generation to the next.

One of the greatest human challenges is how difficult we can make things for ourselves (and the rest of the natural world) when we try to control rather than accept, understand, and cultivate—when we are driven by our amygdala rather than our prefrontal cortex—thereby making us less trustworthy and influential, and therefore less powerful.

As humans, we tend to learn best by doing, to develop and reinforce our neuropathways—by playing, practicing, creating, experimenting, or simulating—which is also why history tends to repeat itself. As humans, we often have to experience something ourselves to really learn from it (even when it's the same mistake others have made and warned us about, especially if we don't trust the person who's warning us).

Due to how the human brain works and learns from repeated behaviors and emotional reinforcement, second-hand knowledge is rarely as powerful as first-hand experiences, which is why we often learn best by doing or experimenting, to learn from trial and error. Since wisdom comes from experience, it's always easier to give advice than it is to take it—to share the lessons we learned from our own first-hand experience, than it is to learn from the experiences of someone else second-hand.

Therefore, human mistakes and imperfection must be

expected, accepted, and embraced as part of the learning and growing process.

Emotional growth, healing, and development all involve the process of learning, whether from your own life experiences, successes, and mistakes or someone else's—through the power of empathy.

Since empathy is powered by our prefrontal cortex that becomes inhibited when stressed, and our long-term memory is directly connected to our unconscious emotional stress response, it can be hard to learn from the mistakes of others when it doesn't trigger a stress response in us—and history repeats itself, time and again. In order for an experience to embed in our own long-term memory, we often have to experience it (or witness it) for ourselves, with our own unconscious emotional stress response to burn it into our long-term memory (lesson learned).

When we ignore or devalue the wisdom of humans who learned before us "the hard way" (by burning the experience into their long-term memory), we set ourselves up to have to learn the hard way ourselves.

Wise humans rely on the knowledge of those who lived before them, so they can live longer, stay safer, travel further, and learn more, thereby advancing the knowledge and lives of those born after them.

And thank goodness for that, or else every generation would have to rediscover how to start a fire, fish and farm, weave and sew, build and construct, manufacture and produce, fly and drive, compute and automate, prevent disaster and disease, and improve health and well-being.

That said, we've still only discovered a fraction of what there is to learn and discover in life, with so much more hidden beneath the surface, to optimize our well-being that includes maintaining a healthy brain, body, and environment.

So consider it an indication of your own wisdom that you are learning from what others before you have explored and discovered, to apply what they learned to your own life, to build on it and teach others how to apply what you learn and discover, to help them feel and do their best.

It might be hard to fathom, but every word you are reading right now, at one time did not exist, and meant absolutely nothing. What started as grunts, groans, lines, and dots eventually evolved into the sounds, symbols, letters, and words we use today. Different groups of humans gave different meanings to different sounds and symbols through the neurological process of repetition and reinforcement that created the collective habit we now call language.

These sounds and symbols became an important way to inform and identify ourselves with a sort of code, to share information or warn others of potential dangers or threats, including other humans, especially those who did not share our communal code. To this day, that code continues to evolve as it passes from one generation to the next, advancing and evolving as it's used more and more with different meaning, or dying off, as it's used less and less.

Shared languages led to the sharing of knowledge and experiences that led to shared systems and beliefs, creating different cultures and identities based on those who shared the same language, knowledge, systems, beliefs, and experiences. Systems of education were then created by humans, based on these languages, to share human knowledge and experiences from one human or group of humans to another.

There are approximately 7,000 languages spoken in the world today, with around twenty of those making up the majority of languages spoken worldwide, with the rest being very rare or dying out from lack of use. There are as many distinct cultures, identities, religions, philosophies, tribes, countries, governments, laws, and cities with different industries, jobs, tools, weapons, styles, social norms, currencies, media, music, games, sports, entertainment, academics, dwellings, healthcare practices, food sources, technologies, etc. Pretty much everything you interact with every moment of every day was created by humans for humans to influence what you do, say, and consume, very often in unconscious ways, and very often in unhealthful ways too.

We all have innate survival instincts that are part of our unconscious stress response to survive the threats we face, be it dangerous weather, wild animals, food scarcity, illness, injury, or attack by other humans. To maintain your brain health and mental well-being, it's important to be aware of these unconscious influences in order to manage your unconscious stress response, to navigate your life in a healthful way, to feel and do your best.

Part of our unconscious mental stress response is our need to understand what threatens us in order to control, avoid, or eliminate the threat. When we feel we have control, our stress response is reduced; and when we feel we have little control, our stress response is heightened, especially when we don't know or trust whoever or whatever is threatening us. As a way to mitigate our stress response, we might unconsciously fill in the gaps of what we don't know (or assume) with what we perceive or believe to be true, in order to have a greater sense of understanding and control.

Have you ever been accused of something you didn't do? This is due to the accuser's unconscious stress response that craves resolve and control of the situation. When we accuse someone of something based on an assumption or perception of what we believe to be true, the critical thinking powers of our prefrontal cortex are inhibited by our unconscious stress response. When our stress response is triggered, it's neurologically easier to blame someone we perceive as a threat to ease our own stress response, rather than admitting we're mistaken or don't know, that could heighten our unconscious stress response with the unknown threat still out there.

As a result of our unconscious stress response, we humans tend to have an unconscious drive to control people, resources, and our environment, including ourselves and each other (with common phrases like, "Control yourself!"). We find relief by trusting and following those who seem in control, who seem to know and understand what threatens us, who we consider our leaders for the sense of safety and control they provide.

Identifying with others who share our language and beliefs provides that sense of trust and safety that every human seeks, that we tend to sense among those who share a common goal (or enemy) for survival.

Thanks to our ability to learn, translate, and share information with others in different ways, we live in a world that knows a bit more each day than it did before. Thanks to our ability to share our knowledge and experience, we don't have to repeat the same mistakes or start from scratch every time a new human is born or a wise one dies (if only we used it as much to share wisdom of hope and healing as dangers and threats!).

While we tend to worry about what we don't know (including the future), we can also prepare for the inevitable twists and turns in life that we can't see around the corner, by practicing how we communicate and navigate the bumps, troubles, and turbulence of life.

Simply put, that's just how the human brain works. Though often misunderstood, underestimated, and overlooked, your brain is a very real neurological and physiological organ that can't just be disregarded or dismissed with an archaic nursery rhyme—no matter how strong, unaffected, and invincible we may want to appear. The only way to truly strengthen your brain and unconscious stress response is to exercise it, not ignore it.

In the same regard, another amazing thing about the human brain is how thoughts and words actually do help us strengthen and heal neurologically and physiologically, in the way that affirmations of love, compassion, and support impact our neurology and physiology.

The challenge, of course, is how much easier it is to remember, repeat, and reinforce those harsh or threatening criticisms, than those loving, supportive, and life affirming messages. Again, we have our human brain to thank for that, since our unconscious stress response is triggered by our amygdala, that is directly connected to our long-term memory, through our sympathetic nervous system. Since the neurological pathways that non-threatening messages take are different, they must be processed consciously through our prefrontal cortex, using repetition of our short-term working memory, to neurologically reinforce them into our long-term memory.

This is the power purpose of conscious effort, practice, and exercise—including repeating positive affirmations—to build and strengthen those healthful neuropathways consciously, to reduce your unconscious stress response and promote a more healthful neurochemical balance, to help you feel and do your best.

Whether you prefer to talk, write, or express your feelings and experiences in other ways, it's important to have a conscious outlet to process them in a healthy way. Those thoughts and feelings in your brain are simply abstract and largely unconscious neurochemical signals until you bring them into your conscious and express them, often through your words, after which you can better understand and manage your own mental and emotional state.

FLEXIBILITY

Level Two: Flexibility

☐ **Get creative without worry of imperfection**

☐ **Practice gratitude to reduce stress and find hope**

☐ **Try something new to stimulate your brain**

☐ **Play a game for the fun and challenge of it**

The practice of flexibility is all about preventing pain and injury, by increasing your resilience and adaptability.

When something is rigid and inflexible, it is more likely to snap, crack, or pop. When it isn't able to bend or respond to stress, pressure, and change in a stabilizing way, it isn't able to maintain its integrity, strength, form, and function.

In humans, this doesn't just happen at the visible physical level, but also the invisible neurological and cellular levels.

When your bones and muscles are more rigid, they are more likely to break or tear. Likewise, if your digestive system has never been challenged to adapt to different foods and nutrients, it's more likely to cause pain, irritation, and indigestion when those new foods and nutrients are introduced. The same goes for your immune system as well. If your immune system is never challenged to adapt and build resilience at the cellular level, it is more vulnerable to illness and disease.

When it comes to physical stretching and weightlifting, you know it's not safe or healthful to just jump into the splits or pick up the heaviest weight in the room without proper preparation. Just as you must slowly stretch to increase your flexibility to the point at which you can safely do the splits, the same goes for your skeletal system, your digestive system, your immune system, and your mental system as well. Never is it healthful to maintain a stressed state without allowing your brain or body to return to a relaxed state to achieve homeostasis, to properly rest, repair, and recover, that is an essential part of the adaption process we call fitness.

It's important to understand the cellular building blocks of your brain and body to practice proper care and preparation.

The neurological and physiological functions of your brain must be safely and healthfully stretched, challenged, and exercised the same way, to maintain resilience and adaptability—to navigate change and challenge, to achieve homoeostasis and return back to a less stressed state.

Similar to physical challenges, it can feel uncomfortable when your thought patterns are challenged because of the neurochemical process involved.

Your neuropathways are actual pathways that have been blazed through your brain like a trail through a forest, with repetition and reinforcement. When you're first learning or blazing the trail, it takes a lot of work and effort; but over time, the pathways become clearer and stronger, allowing you to pass faster and more easily to get where you want to go with little thought or effort.

When you're suddenly forced to redirect and find another pathway to get where you want to go, you are suddenly challenged to leave the path you had forged, to find a new one, that takes time, energy, and intention to forge again—with repetition and reinforcement, that requires motivation and reward, and a sense of hope.

At first, you might resist leaving the existing pathway, since it is the one you have always used. With repeated use, it forged clearly and deeply in your brain, and energy passed quickly and easily, with little effort. At one time it provided hope, motivation, and reward, but no longer does. Accepting this new reality can be very painful and challenging, due to the rush of neurochemicals flowing without clear direction, in an effort to forge new neuropathways to achieve a similar result that may be impossible or at least extremely difficult, without a stress-reducing sense of hope or reward.

Can you imagine waking up tomorrow to find your car was stolen, a loved one had died, your house was destroyed, or you could no longer walk, talk, hear, or see?

Of course none of us like to think about any of these highly stress-inducing scenarios that trigger an extreme stress response, but it's also a part of practicing flexibility in order to develop resilience. While you certainly shouldn't dwell or worry about the possibility of loss and tragedy (that could result in a sustained stressful state that may contribute to or exacerbate anxiety, depression, or other mental health conditions), being mentally prepared for the worst-case scenario, while hoping for the best-case scenario, can be a healthful way to practice navigating stress with mental flexibility.

When you finally accept that the pathway no longer gets you where you want to go, or that the place that used to bring you a sense of joy, love, safety, and comfort no longer exists, you feel lost and hopeless—much like feeling lost and hopeless in the woods—triggering a stress response of fear, anxiety, anger, and depression, that we know as grief.

Like the rest of your body, your brain is more relaxed and at ease when things are easy, that requires less energy and effort; and feels stressed when faced with a threat, change, or challenge, that requires energy and effort.

However, just because a person, situation, or other life change challenges your brain, does not make it a real threat or enemy, even when it might feel that way. Either way, your unconscious stress response is triggered by perceived threats, until your prefrontal cortex can analyze and determine the situation as safe and healthful, with your powers of critical thinking and comprehension.

For example, when someone disagrees with you, it does not mean they are threatening your life or harming you. Sometimes when presented with conflicting information or a different perspective, it might actually contribute to your health and well-being, as an opportunity for learning and growth.

The challenge is engaging your brain in a way that allows you to know the difference, and it can be hard to tell the difference when we're not provided a safe or supportive environment— when others might even be criticizing and shaming you in the process (that increases your stress response rather than reducing it).

The practice of flexibility is intended to challenge thoughts and feelings, without being told what to think and feel.

Practicing compassion, empathy, and forgiveness in moments of stress is an essential practice to healthfully manage and reduce your stress response by activating and energizing your higher functioning prefrontal cortex.

Flexibility is an important part of adaptation and resilience that takes time and patience, with progressive incremental challenges as well as stress relief. You can start with a small amount of stress, like being creative or playing a game, and build up to a larger amount of stress, like preparing for the worst-case scenario, while hoping for the best-case scenario. As with any flexibility practice, remember to include periods of rest and recovery in between moments of stress, to allow healthful adaptation.

The healthful aim is never to make people feel uncomfortable for the sake of making them uncomfortable, but to help people work through discomfort to feel more comfortable, stronger, and better off, even when it may be uncomfortable to start. We feel discomfort for a reason, and it's important to know why, to understand ourselves and each other better.

21 CREATIVITY AND IMAGINATION

Have you attempted to bake something from scratch without using a recipe? Have you invented or created something that nobody had before?

If so, then you know the power of trial and error, and practicing mental flexibility!

The important lessons you can learn through creativity and exploration often lead to new ideas, better understanding, and even better outcomes. By accepting mistakes and imperfections, you may even discover something you didn't intend to make or that you like even more than what you originally had in mind!

Lifelong learning and practice are essential to mental fitness. The best kind of education is often one that embraces imperfection and allows you to accept that you don't know it all, that life is full of mysteries, and that it's OK to ask questions.

To our detriment, we're often taught that ignorance and imperfection are "bad," to be rejected, denied, or avoided. We become afraid of looking stupid, or fear that someone will use our ignorance or imperfection against us to reduce our power and influence. So sometimes we fake it, or convince ourselves that we know when we really don't—inhibiting the opportunity to learn, explore, and discover.

This fear can manifest into jealousy of others who achieve and succeed. We can feel bad about ourselves when we compare ourselves to others, without knowing the stress, practice, failed attempts, criticisms, or learning process that took place before they achieved and succeeded. Our sense of jealousy can become toxic when we use it to tear others down for their successes and achievements, because we are also unconsciously reinforcing our own fear of being criticized and torn down for our own achievements and successes—perpetuating an unconscious fear of both failure and success (making it even harder to just get started).

No, this isn't because you or anyone else is a jerk or an evil person. It's just how the human brain works that must be understood in order to improve healthful brain function and performance.

Since we don't know what we don't know, our brains tend to unconsciously fill in the blanks based on what we do know, including our own experiences and unconscious biases.

For example, when you look at a photo or watch a video clip, what do you imagine beyond the frame?

Do you imagine the scene continuing all around and behind the camera, or do you imagine the set, lighting, and camera crew?

This is an example of the power of magic and illusion that any good magician (or advertising professional) knows, based on the powers of your perception. Your brain is continuously unconsciously filling in the blanks between the bits and pieces of sensory information you process to form a more complete mental picture and sense of understanding.

A whole fantastical world of magical beings and mythical beasts can be created in your head by hearing or reading a few words, or seeing a picture or drawing. Your brain unconsciously perceives that actors are actually feeling the feelings they feel, that stimulate your unconscious emotions too, even when you consciously know they are just pretending.

Your brain completes the picture with the power of your imagination that can either work for or against you. You can believe that someone else has it all—perceiving life as perfect, care-free, and easy (the mythical appeal of being "rich and famous")—because of what you don't know; or you can use your powers of imagination and creativity to explore, learn, innovate, and entertain, by imagining an alternate reality or possibilities to explore.

When attempting to create something from scratch, an empty space, page, or canvas can seem frightening and intimidating, due to our fear of failure (or success) that inhibits us from getting started. It can be less intimidating to start with something than nothing, so my mental fitness tip is to start by putting something in that blank space, however imperfect or undeveloped. You can always change it as you go, which is the whole point of practicing creativity to develop mental flexibility. It's important to remember that there's no need for perfection or rigidity, especially at the beginning of something new.

So what does "perfect" mean to you? Do you strive to be perfect? Does perfection mean meeting the demands and expectations of others, or your own?

How does the desire to be perfect affect you? Does it bring out the best or the worst in you?

Does striving for perfection make you feel more or less creative and successful?

Once you achieve perfection, what's next?

It seems once we do achieve perfection (however we define it), we're expected to maintain and repeat it. This is why it's often said, "No good deed goes unpunished." After you achieve a goal or succeed at something, the expectation (or metaphorical bar) is often for you to repeat that achievement over and over again, without realizing the unhealthy impact.

To do something perfectly once is a great achievement (based on whatever characteristics qualify it as "perfect"), but the expectation to continually "be perfect" or that perfection should be sustained indefinitely also creates a continuous level of stress that is not healthful.

This is why Olympic athletes who train for years to perform perfectly often experience a state of depression after the Olympics are over, with that sudden drop in energizing neurochemicals that once fueled their motivation. Those who plan for years to have the "perfect wedding" may also experience a state of depression after their wedding day for the same reason, that sudden crash in neurochemicals.

When we have "perfection" as a goal, we often experience states of depression and anxiety as well, but may be too afraid to share it since our fear of failure is so intense. The stress we put on ourselves to be "perfect" is a way to unconsciously mask our unconscious emotions, to avoid conscious awareness by using stress to fuel our motivation with a high level of adrenaline and cortisol to prevent that neurochemical crash.

The biggest problem with "perfection" is that it doesn't allow for failure, experimentation, or exploration, which is often when we discover and learn the most.

What is "perfect" is also completely subjective based on one's perception, taste, and preference. What is perfect to one may not be perfect to another if they don't feel the same sense of pleasure or benefits from it (which makes the word "perfect" seem a bit imperfect itself).

Have you ever tried to play matchmaker by pairing one friend with another who you think would be perfect for each other based on your perception of them, only to find they don't like each other that way? (Awk-ward.)

Or maybe your perfect lunch is a peanut butter sandwich, while that same exact sandwich you love to eat could actually kill someone else who is allergic to peanuts.

Yet we often expect others to like what we like and are often baffled when others don't like the things we do. Even worse, we tend to take it personally, as though their dislike of what we like means they don't like us as a person, that triggers our stress response. You might feel bad or even mad. Your emotions might trigger a defensive reaction by shaming them for not liking what you like, or for liking something you don't. You might even perceive them as an enemy instead of a friend.

Sometimes what might seem like the most trivial and insignificant things, like personal taste and preferences, can feel uncomfortable and divisive due to our unconscious stress response. Without emotional awareness or awareness of what influences our mental functions, we are more likely to perceive that anything or anyone that makes us feel bad is bad, and is something or someone to avoid. It's this unconscious stress response that can impair your growth, healing, and learning when you avoid things that trigger your stress response and challenge you to examine your feelings that make you afraid of conflict and being hurt again—that makes you more rigid and less flexible.

Goals and expectations are definitely important for motivation and achievement (especially for high-risk jobs), but goals and expectations must also be realistic and achievable to avoid unhealthy outcomes. We must be realistic about the possibility and sustainability to properly prepare our brain to maintain neurological health, well-being, and performance.

That goes for your fitness practice too—the most intimidating part is just getting started without trying to be perfect!

We are all growing, learning, developing, and adapting as we go, and need to be granted the time, space, and freedom from perfection to do so. After that, every step can feel like an achievement, when you're allowed to feel your best to do your best.

So when faced with the dread of imperfection, or you don't believe you're creative, remember that achievement isn't always at the end, and creativity isn't always about the product, but the process. There is achievement in feeling, doing, creating, and growing as you go. The most important part is that you just get started, and keep going.

22 GRATITUDE AND EMPATHY

Why do we tend to take what we have for granted—like our health, family, friends, life, safety, security, or just feeling fine—and waste so much conscious energy focused on what we don't have?

Why do we value what's rare or difficult to obtain and take for granted what comes easily to us (that might even be rare or difficult for someone else)?

Most of your emotions are actually unconscious neurochemical responses that require no conscious effort or awareness.

Therefore, when what you have no longer triggers that rush of neurochemicals that comes from anticipation and excitement, we tend to think that what we have is boring or not enough.

Do you remember that thing you were so desperate and excited to have, and how quickly that excitement wore off after you got it?

How many things did you absolutely love when you first got them to only lose interest shortly after?

Due to how our human brains work, it's only after we lose something and experience the unconscious neurochemical stress response of loss, when we realize how rare and precious what we had was (whether our health, family, friends, home, pet, etc.), and how much joy and happiness what we had actually brought us—even when our unconscious neurochemicals didn't react as such.

You deserve to be happy, but happiness doesn't always come easily, especially when our unconscious brain is on the constant lookout for problems and reasons to be unhappy. Sacrificing your own happiness to make someone else happy is not healthful, and that sort of power dynamic is actually toxic and abusive. When one can only be happy when the other is happy, the influence that one has over the other is considered a form of codependency, that can be extremely stressful, inhibiting, and unhealthy.

The pursuit of happiness requires conscious effort to calm your amygdala to find the joys in life that includes practicing gratitude. Practicing gratitude is a way to consciously elicit good feeling that you no longer unconsciously feel when what you have is no longer new or exciting, and no longer elicits your unconscious emotional response.

Unless you're reading this in a sensory deprivation tank, there are likely sights, sounds, sensations, and even smells that you are not consciously aware of, until you make a conscious effort to notice them. Stop for a moment and be consciously aware of them. What do you hear? What do you smell? How do you feel? This is your reality that your brain is unconsciously processing, but you may not be consciously aware. Take this moment to feel consciously grateful for your life, your breath, your abilities, and what you have in this moment.

Your unconscious brain is constantly absorbing many more bits of sensory information that go unnoticed and forgotten

215

until they trigger your unconscious stress response (zapping your amygdala), or you focus your conscious attention on them (with your prefrontal cortex). Fragments of these unconscious experiences remain in your unconscious mind, which is why certain sounds, smells, sensations, or visual cues may trigger a memory or unconscious emotional response.

While empathy is most often thought of in terms of relating to another's pain or loss, it's also important to practice empathy to relate to another's pride and joy. The ability to feel happiness in another's happiness is one quick way to increase your own level of happiness to feel more grateful and socially connected, to reduce your unconscious stress response. When practiced properly, empathy is an important mental fitness practice that supports neurological growth and development as well.

Since we can only ever experience life from our own perspective, there remains a lot that we don't know about life from the perspectives and experiences of other people. It's practically impossible to describe our lived experience in every possible detail to someone else. There is so much to our lived experience that others will never truly know; but thanks to our powers of imagination and empathy, we can at least give others a taste of our lived experience by sharing through spoken or written word, or visually through illustration, painting, video, or photography.

The best we can do is tap into our empathic abilities by engaging our prefrontal cortex—that functions best when we aren't otherwise stressed, and may also be more challenging to do for those with a neurological or development difference—. Empathy involves listening, learning, and sharing lived experiences to give ourselves a sort of emotional taste of another person's lived experience, by using our imagination to consider their perspective, thoughts, and feelings rather than just our own.

It's important to note that while empathy is an important brain function, it can also trigger our unconscious stress response when the feelings and experiences we empathize with are stressful ones. For this reason, highly empathetic people may be more susceptible to developing anxiety and depression when conscious activity triggers their unconscious stress response. It's like a mental storm when neurons fire back and forth between your prefrontal cortex and your amygdala, resulting in a perpetual state of stress.

Since our unconscious neurological activity happens faster than we can even consciously assess our feelings, emotional regulation can be that much harder when we don't give our brain a break. When the neurological storm of anxiety gets too strong, it might also result in a panic attack, memory loss, or other health conditions when our unconscious stress response overwhelms our neurological and physiological system.

This is why it's important to practice getting "out of your head." While you can't literally get out of your own head, you can practice focusing your conscious attention on something outside of you by doing something creative, moving your body, looking at nature, or even volunteering and helping others. By focusing your conscious attention on something other than the thoughts swimming in your head, you can also help calm the neurological storm to navigate in more healthful ways.

Imagination and storytelling play a critical role in the practice of empathy too. By consciously listening or imagining how someone else feels, including their joys, pains, struggles, and achievements, you can develop a greater sense of acceptance and understanding.

It's important to differentiate empathy from sympathy as well. Sympathy often relates to the sense of pity or sorrow we feel when our mind remains in a third-person perspective, and the emotions we feel stem from our own experience.

For example, if someone dies of a painful disease, you might sympathize with their loved ones for their loss based on how you feel about death and loss. You may not empathize with the complexity of their emotions, however, unless you can imagine the emotional complexity of experiencing both grief and relief at the same time—grieving the loss of a loved one while simultaneously feeling relieved that they are no longer suffering in pain.

Similarly, you might feel sympathy for someone who seems to have less than you—whether in health, wealth, relationships, or abilities—for how dreadful you feel it would be to not have what you have. Empathy, on the other hand, considers their feelings, experiences, values, and beliefs that may differ from your own, and how much pride and joy they feel with the health, wealth, relationships, or abilities they do have, regardless of what others have.

When we rely on feeling pity for others in order to feel grateful for what we have, we risk contributing to a toxic social hierarchy in which we unconsciously keep others down in order to lift ourselves up. This is why practicing empathy for other's joys, successes, and achievements is just as important as practicing empathy for their pain, loss, and struggles—to maintain a healthful balance.

Of course, we cannot actually experience someone else's experiences first-hand, neurologically or physiologically, which is why even when we empathize, we are still limited to our own imagination and mental abilities (which is also why empathy may be harder for some than others, depending on their neurological state and development). While we might imagine their feelings and experiences, nothing can take the place of the person who actually lived and experienced them, which is why diversity and inclusion are so important, to represent and share the diverse lived experiences and perspectives of every individual.

23 COURAGE AND CURIOSITY

What does courage mean to you?

While courage is often defined as taking action in the face of fear, it's really much more than that. Sometimes the most courageous thing you can do is calmly stand your ground, or calmly walk away.

Courage is the practice of relaxing the unconscious stress response of your amygdala enough to engage the higher functions of your prefrontal cortex, including comprehension, critical thinking, emotional regulation, problem solving, empathy, and impulse control—that requires conscious effort.

We sometimes call it "hot headed" when our amygdala is triggered and drives our behavior, or "cool headed" when the prefrontal cortex is engaged to calm our unconscious stress response.

The practice of courage can be harder for some than others depending on brain health, experience, and neurological state, which is why it's a practice that must be healthfully repeated and reinforced.

It takes courage to not let your fears get the best of you (including your health), and to help others do the same.

Courage is the ability to not react impulsively (driven by your amygdala), but responding in a healthful way that achieves a healthful outcome (driven by your prefrontal cortex).

For example, which do you consider more courageous? Impulsively kicking a dog that growls at you because you're afraid of it, or choosing to work at an animal shelter to overcome your fear of dogs?

Courage isn't just fighting instead of fleeing or freezing, or attacking what or who you fear impulsively with that rush of cortisol and adrenaline triggered by your amygdala.

Courage is your ability to be aware of your feelings to navigate them in a healthful way, to achieve a healthful outcome.

Whatever you fear, courage is your ability to use the power of your conscious mind to navigate your unconscious stress response in the heat of the moment, that requires conscious effort and practice.

Courage is the ability to better manage your fear and stress response, rather than letting your fear or stress response control you.

Understanding your fears and what drives them is an important mental fitness exercise as well, to help you feel and do your best. It's also probably one of the most uncomfortable, since it "pokes the bear" in your brain that is your amygdala.

A major part of promoting brain health and mental fitness is awareness of unhealthy influences that contribute to an unhealthy level of stress in your system, and where they come from—whether socially, environmentally, nutritionally, or chemically.

Fear tactics are often used to inhibit the higher powers of your prefrontal cortex by continuously triggering your unconscious stress response—to influence your thoughts, feelings, and behaviors. Practicing courage by consciously navigating your unconscious stress response is a healthful way to build resilience against these manipulative fear tactics.

Staying away from what you are afraid of may be the most healthful response in the short-term, but in the long-term—when those fears are debilitating and preventing you from living your best life—facing your fears when you are able and ready may be the only way to learn, grow, and thrive.

We often equate emotional strength with courage, to not be afraid of the unknown or our ignorance, to constantly ask questions and even question authority, to attempt to do something you've never attempted to do before.

If emotional strength is characterized by courage, then we're probably the strongest as infants—before we learn to be afraid of failure, afraid of what we don't know, afraid of pain and what might harm us. Even when we're toddlers, we constantly question authority by asking, "Why?" until the authority figure runs out of answers or patience (an emotional strength), and turns blue in the face, with their head feeling like it's about to explode (i.e., their stress response).

We're often taught that curiosity killed the cat as a lesson to ask questions or be curious, when it's really ignorance that killed that cat because it didn't know better.

In this regard, curiosity is a form of courage.

Curiosity leads to learning that leads to knowledge, which leads to the wisdom of knowing better, that can also reduce fear, stress, and biases (driven by the amygdala) by promoting critical thinking and problem solving (driven by the prefrontal cortex).

Curiosity can actually promote safety, healing, and well-being by promoting learning and comprehension, and reducing our unconscious fear and stress response that can get in the way.

In reality, ignorance is NOT bliss when we don't know better, and our unconscious stress response makes us too afraid to learn or explore, or experience something new that can help us grow, heal, and thrive.

So for your own health and well-being, stay curious.

As kids, we're dreamers and doers, and the future is full of opportunity. We find motivation in all that is fun, mysterious, and challenging, especially when we receive praise for trying. It's only when the reward of trying wears off that we only find pleasure in the reward of succeeding, or winning, that changes us in two ways—we feel motivated when we perceive a chance of success or winning, and unmotivated when we don't (reinforcing our fear of failure, when we no longer allow ourselves to learn through trial and error).

If you feel you're not happy enough, tall enough, thin enough, funny enough, sexy enough, sensitive enough, tough enough, strong enough, successful enough, rich enough, white enough, black enough, masculine enough, feminine enough, or whatever other value judgment we place on ourselves and each other that trigger our unconscious stress response in an attempt to control and manipulate thoughts, feelings, and behaviors—the most important lesson to learn is that you ARE enough, no matter what.

You deserve to feel and do your best as much as anyone else, even when how you feel and what you can do might differ.

We are all born with needs that continue through life, including adequate time, care, safety, and nutrition, from the moment we are conceived, until our dying day, that requires adequate resources and support along the way. There's no "secret" in that.

One of the biggest challenges is realizing what kind of support you need when you need it, and having the courage to seek it, ask for it, and find it. Knowing who and how to ask is the real trick.

If you have a goal, share it with others. Tell those who will encourage and support you, to help you maintain your hope and motivation.

Optimism and positive thinking are powerful neurological influences that help you stay hopeful and motivated neurologically as well. Your healthful energy and example can also be perceived by others in your attitude, behaviors, and body language. Those who feel inspired by your ambition, optimism, and positivity (and don't feel threatened by it) will feel motivated to support you too. You'll likely appreciate their help so much that you'll feel motivated to help them in return!

That's the power of being a healthful influence ourselves, when we influence and motivate each other in healthful ways. Society is an ecosystem, and we reap what we sow.

24 WORK AND BUSINESS

What influences your level of stress, your expectations, and your sense of control?

We all want a sense of control (even when we actually have very little control), because when we don't, we feel like we're being controlled, limited, and inhibited, that triggers an unconscious stress response.

Other animals do not flourish in captivity, and neither do humans. We resort to captivity and isolation as a form of punishment in an attempt to influence behaviors through concession and conformity, but in doing so, we often fail to engage the all-important prefrontal cortex in a healthful way, to heal the root cause of the unhealthy behavior that's likely driven by unconscious emotion.

One big benefit of being self-employed is choosing a title that reflects your responsibilities. A title may seem insignificant, but it influences both your self-perception and the perception others have of you. When you're self-employed, you can practically change your title every day to best fit your evolving role, services, and responsibilities.

In corporate America, however, this is not often the case. While responsibilities often change and get reassigned, titles seem more static and difficult to change, since title is often associated with seniority and pay grade, all regimented and systematized.

Perception of self can be a real barrier to job satisfaction and a contributor to attrition as well, when one's title and pay doesn't reflect the actual value of the work they do, that impacts their self-esteem and self-worth. This stems more from how a person feels doing the work than the actual work itself, whether they feel adequately recognized, respected, and rewarded—whether they neurologically experience repetition with reinforcement, or just repetition without reinforcement.

Anxiety can also drain your confidence and motivation, and deteriorate your health and happiness. It can literally feel like a mental storm in your head that you can't control, that just makes you want to run and hide. I constantly worried how others perceived and judged me (and still do, thankfully to a lesser extent), which is why managing anxiety is a big part of my own mental fitness practice.

It wasn't until later in life when I learned about brain function in practical terms, when I was better able to manage it, with knowledge of how stress triggers the amygdala and inhibits the prefrontal cortex, and how mental health conditions are also related to many physical health conditions, neurologically and physiologically. I was never taught any of this in health or science classes, and had to learn the hard way by experiencing and researching on my own (that might be why you're reading this book too!).

Mental health issues don't just go away with a wish or a happy thought. Whether mental or physical, maintaining your fitness, health, and well-being takes proper care and continual effort.

It can help to push yourself out of your comfort zone at times, to challenge and develop your perceptions in healthier ways, to reduce the unconscious stress response of perceived threats. Similar to setting physical fitness goals, my mental fitness goals have included singing in a band, speaking in public for fundraisers and community service events, leading businesses, and attending many networking events. Out of all, it's actually networking that I find to be the most challenging, since it requires so much conscious energy to manage my unconscious stress response with each and every new person I meet.

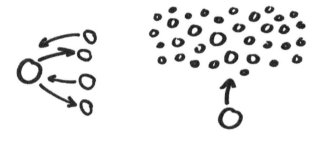

I actually find performing or speaking in front of a crowd (or even staffing an information table) a lot less anxiety-inducing than networking a room full of people. When I perceive the audience as one group, or I can remain in one spot and have people come to me for information, my anxiety is at a much lower level than when I walk into a room full of people, with whom I must network, when I struggle to even know where or how to begin (that induces my anxiety).

Is networking, performing, or public speaking a source of anxiety or strength for you?

What makes you feel like you have limited time, energy, and resources?

It's important to remember that it's not just businesses that benefit from saving time, money, and resources, but also YOU.

Wealth isn't just accumulated by making more money but also saving it by spending less—so improving your health can also improve your wealth—by reducing stress that allows you to think more critically and creatively, to make wiser and healthier choices.

Using your time, energy, and resources in an efficient and effective way also means that you can save time, money, and resources.

You will never be able to add more hours to the day, or squeeze blood from a penny; but if you spend your time, energy, and resources wisely on those things that reduce stress, and support your health and well-being, you'll have more time, energy, and resources to spare!

Even when you are encouraged to spend every ounce of your time, energy, and resources to benefit someone else—with whatever promise they make as a reward for your sacrifice—the greatest reward is more time, energy, and resources, because they are all limited. That is why so many people sacrifice all they have for fame and fortune, with the promise of happiness (the danger of high expectations), and so often end up unhappy when they realize all the time and energy they sacrificed, with little left to actually enjoy.

No amount of money can ever buy back the time or energy that you already spent, which is why it's so important to spend it wisely, and healthfully.

Your stress will not be reduced by a bigger house, fancier cars, gourmet foods, or luxury vacations—especially if you can't find the time to schedule it, and aren't able to disconnect from the stress when you're on it. Again, you might get a neurochemical rush of dopamine when you purchase something new and fancy, as a reward and excitement like a dream come true, but the original stress you had that earned you the cash you used to buy these things remains—and now you've set a higher mental expectation for yourself that will make it harder for your brain to feel excited to get that rush of dopamine next time (with a bigger house to clean and repair, and a more expensive car to maintain too).

The only good that money can actually do is pay for what you need, including the necessary help and support you need to reduce stress and improve your health and well-being, whether in the form of support staff, childcare, senior care, training, coaching, therapy, or other form of care and support.

If clinical mental health services are not covered by your benefits, your request is a valid one, and will help build a business case for it.

Supplemental services like mental fitness programs might also provide an affordable preventive care option by promoting healthful practices that promote brain health and mental well-being, which can be used in combination with clinical health services.

Lastly, if you run a business, put people first by providing the care and support they need.

Any successful business knows that people are not disposable parts that can just be used and replaced when they wear out. Businesses that put profit before people, and neglect the health and well-being of their employees, put their business at risk, by failing to invest in the health and vitality of their human capital.

I have a hard time thinking of any job (whether paid or volunteer) that is absolutely stress-free, because that in essence is the value of our work—the value of our time and energy to help solve a problem or meet a demand (i.e., stress).

There is a difference between the stress of working hard to

provide for yourself and your family that benefits your health and well-being, versus the stress of not getting time off to rest and replenish your health and well-being. Every brain and body requires rest in order to recover and rebalance. As humans, we are innately social animals, who benefit from social support, that is the power of community, and a healthful level of interdependence that provides relief, encouragement, and support when we need it, to avoid being crushed by the weight (i.e., stressors) of life on our own.

With all of this "unhealthy" talk about the neurological and physiological effects of stress, stress is also an important and unavoidable part of life that can have healthful effects, in healthful amounts, when you're able to use it to achieve healthful outcomes. When you're in a stressed state, and you're able to use your conscious mind to regulate your emotions and impulses, all of your mental energy is used to get hyper-focused on that one threat or stress—maybe it's a final exam, a public speech, or a serious debate.

The practice of avoiding or "drowning out" distractions in these moments is important, since paying attention to other distractions takes your focus and energy away from the threat or stress you are trying to focus on, further triggering your unconscious stress response, inhibiting your conscious focus, and impairing your performance. This is why "multitasking" is never as efficient or effective as focusing on one task at a time, and why you might get irritated or angered by distractions when you're trying to focus. You might even turn down the radio or tell others to be quiet when you're in a stressful driving situation, to reduce your unconscious stress response and increase your conscious attention on the situation.

There's nothing you can do to not have any stress at all in your life. Without any stress, humans would never evolve or adapt. Life would actually feel quite boring and meaningless with nothing to challenge you or give you that rewarding sense of achievement after accomplishing a challenging goal or difficult task.

As animals, we often need that sense of stress to provide a sense of direction (toward safety), purpose (to seek safety), and accomplishment (to find safety) to keep moving, growing, and thriving in life. A sense of excitement or anticipation is another form stress that stimulates a similar, but different, combination of neurochemicals than those stimulated by fear and danger. Your sympathetic nervous system is stimulated to promote blood flow and get your muscles ready for movement and action—which is why we might cheer, jump or do cartwheels! The healthful result of excitement and anticipation is the immense sense of hope that fuels your motivation (rather than fear or panic), that stimulates an immense sense of relief, when the stressful experience ends by meeting or exceeding our expectations—or an immense sense of disappointment with a neurochemical crash, if expectations are not met (the reason to set realistic expectations).

It's how you balance, manage, and navigate the stresses in life that really makes the biggest difference in your health and well-being.

REST & RECOVERY

Level Three: Rest & Recovery

☐ **Get enough quality sleep to detoxify**

☐ **Eat well and hydrate to get the nutrients you need**

☐ **Practice meditation and/or controlled breathing**

☐ **Limit distractions and stressful media**

The practice of rest and recovery is all about prioritizing sleep, self-care, stress reduction, nutrition, and healing that are all essential to human growth and development. Taking time to rest and recover is a vital part of your health and well-being, that often gets dismissed or downplayed in our highly competitive culture, in which there never seem to be enough hours in a day to get everything done that we expect of ourselves, in order to feel like a winner.

As we all navigate the human challenges of life, please practice compassion for yourself and others, and take a break when you need it. Allow your brain the time and space needed to process, rest, refuel, and recover, and know that your feelings are real, natural, and valid neurochemical signals as a neurochemical human being.

25 SLEEP FOR YOUR HEALTH

Getting quality sleep has as much to do with promoting brain health as maintaining your overall physical health, as your metabolic and mental processes work together to detoxify your biological systems while you sleep.

Unfortunately, our highly competitive culture in which "time is money" and "the early bird gets the worm" usually fails to include sleep as a priority—that is even more important than our workload! We have seriously undervalued and underrated the importance of sleep as a culture, including how to maintain a healthful sleep routine that has become a detriment to our health and well-being, as well as our performance and productivity (isn't it ironic, Alanis?).

When you're awake and active, your body and brain produce various byproducts from normal cellular activity throughout the day. Adenosine is one of those byproducts that's produced, which is also one of the chemicals that makes you feel sleepy at the end of the day. This is the neurochemical that is blocked by caffeine to make your brain and body feel more awake—that is, until the caffeine wears off and you have a "caffeine crash" when that buildup of adenosine rushes back to tell your brain

233

and body that you should be sleeping.

During sleep, your brain and body quite literally flush these toxic byproducts (including adenosine) out of your brain and body to rebalance your system, making you feel refreshed and awake. Getting enough sleep to allow enough detoxifying deep sleep cycles (that usually takes around 7-9 hours of quality sleep) is so important to maintaining your health, neurology, and physiology—including healthier skin and organs, by reducing toxic inflammation and optimizing your mental and physical functions!

26 NUTRITION, DRUGS, AND DIGESTION

It's not just a cliché—you absolutely are what you eat. Every cell in your brain and body is made up of the minerals and nutrients that you consume. When you don't get the proper building blocks that your brain and body need to properly maintain, heal, and develop, you will have a harder time feeling and doing your best.

In addition, with so many artificial ingredients and toxic chemicals in what the modern-day human now consumes, the unhealthful reality is that most of us are not getting the essential minerals and nutrients that our brains and body need to optimize function, health, and well-being—which contributes to a number of the physical, mental, emotional, and behavioral health crises we're facing. Your gut plays a critical role in your brain health and mental functions as well, which is why it's important to be aware of what you eat, how you feel, and how to best optimize your nutrition to feel and do your best (often requiring a nutritional supplement if you cannot get enough essential nutrients naturally).

What makes healthful living even more challenging is when people make money off of the very things that harm us. Trying to get rid of the unhealthy things that are often incredibly tempting, accessible, and affordable is an uphill battle, when those things are also the livelihood and source of income for so many people (whether they work in manufacturing, retail, or distribution). It's another self-perpetuating toxic cycle when we're all trying to make money to survive, and the money comes from something that also threatens our health, safety, and survival.

When we don't have the same access to healthful and affordable options, trying to tell people to make healthful choices and change their behaviors is a bit like telling someone to walk up the escalator when the escalator is going down.

Another important fact is that the human brain is made of approximately 75% water, which is why water is essential for healthful brain function as an electrochemical organ.

Alcohol and caffeine can impair healthful brain function and development by dehydrating your system and contributing to other neurochemical and physiological imbalances. While drinking caffeine in moderation may have healthful effects, by increasing alertness and promoting blood flow, it can also have unhealthy effects by triggering anxiety and other health conditions related to neurological and physiological imbalances. Alcohol affects the neurochemical levels of glutamate and GABA in your system, relaxing your muscles and slowing your metabolism, as well as slowing the reaction time of your prefrontal cortex (not to mention the deceptively high level of empty calories that have no nutritional value). It's important to know your own brain and body to know your limits and how much is too much—if any at all.

We are often unconsciously attempting to alter our mental and emotional state to feel better with either caffeine or alcohol that can be a health problem in itself. When we rely on consuming potentially harmful chemicals as a means of altering our mental and emotional state, as a form of self-medicating, that's the time to speak with your healthcare provider. Consuming caffeine and alcohol can actually make the situation worse either by disrupting sleep or inhibiting emotional regulation and impulse control, further contributing to physical, mental, emotional, and behavioral health issues.

There is no shame in drinking caffeine or alcohol, in moderation, for your own enjoyment, when there is no adverse impact on your health or well-being; but it's important to know the health risks so you can be empowered to make the most healthful decisions for yourself.

Don't be fooled by the marketing ploy called "Happy Hour" (especially if it's only masking chronic pain and stress).

Now go drink a happy glass of water. Your brain and body will thank you!

27 MEDITATION

Mental fitness practices are not intended to tell you what to think or believe, but to help you identify the healthful influences you need to develop and maintain healthful habits and behaviors to feel and do your best. Mental fitness practices allow you to explore how and why you think, feel, and behave the way you do, to develop greater conscious awareness of your brain health and mental functions, including unconscious functions, to better manage your overall health and well-being.

The practice of meditation sometimes gets confused as a religious or spiritual practice since various religions and spiritual leaders practice meditation in different ways, including the meditative practice of prayer.

In terms of brain health and mental fitness, meditation is quite simply a mindfulness practice to help calm and balance your nervous system, to help lower those neurochemicals that put wear and tear on your brain and body, and increase the more healthful and healing ones by engaging your parasympathetic nervous system.

You can have a meditative experience just by getting outside and spending time in nature, even if just standing or sitting. It's important to remember that you are a vital part of nature just like every other plant, animal, and element, and to care for yourself just the same. Spending time in nature increases vitamin D from sunlight and oxygen produced by plants and trees that support healthful neurological and physiological activity.

While a calm and quiet place is best for meditating, to calm and relax your mind, you can even do a short meditation in public when you feel your stress level rising.

Closing your eyes and placing your hands on your lap can also help reduce distraction and increase your focus to relax your mind.

Using a word or phrase without meaning while you meditate (otherwise known as a "mantra") can also help calm and focus your mind. If a mantra had meaning, then your mind would naturally think about things related to that word.

All of that said, your mind will still naturally wonder and wander with distractions while you meditate. This wondering and wandering is an important part of the meditation practice, a bit like lifting weights. Every time your mind wanders a bit (like lowering the weight) you gently return your focus back to your breathing or your mantra (like lifting the weight again). The practice should be smooth, gentle, and natural, to strengthen your neurological control just as you would a muscle.

It's called a practice for a reason, since it's a process you repeat again and again to help balance your mind, strengthen your neurological network, and improve your mental dexterity and flexibility.

The point of meditation is essentially to practice calming your unconscious stress response by focusing your conscious mind in a peaceful way, lowering your neurochemical stress to help calm your nervous system throughout your brain and body.

28 TAKE A BREAK FROM DEVICES

For many, the most challenging mental fitness practice may be turning off digital devices and limiting stressful media.

These days, much of our news and entertainment is stress-inducing. We can actually become addicted to media consumption by the neurochemical release triggered by our unconscious stress response, including a rush of adrenaline and dopamine.

That adrenaline rush activates your autonomic nervous system and alters your body chemistry, which is why stress followed by a hit of dopamine (when your stress response is relieved) can be so addictive. So much so, that we actually have names for such conditions like FOMO (fear of missing out) or being an "adrenaline junky."

We might turn to social media in an attempt to relieve our stress, maybe as a form of journaling or chat therapy, but therapy it is not.

You may not feel safe or comfortable sharing or discussing your emotional struggles with others, especially if we fear shame, retaliation, or being perceived as flawed, weak, or incapable.

Of course media is big business and big money, used to advertise as much as entertain, with influential marketing and product placement by psychological design. Media influencers actually get paid for psychologically influencing their followers, getting paid for the number of hits that a post about their product generates.

The media we consume absolutely influences our perceptions, attitudes, and behaviors, fueled by the big money generated from it. It's therefore as important to be a wise consumer of media as much as the food you consume, since it impacts your brain function and mental activity neurologically and physiologically.

When your amygdala triggers a stress response, it sends an immediate electrochemical signal to another part of your brain called your hypothalamus, that in turn unconsciously activates the sympathetic branch of your autonomic nervous system (that automates and regulates bodily functions). This triggers your adrenal glands to release adrenaline into your blood stream to divert energy away from organs like your stomach to give your heart, lungs, and muscles a sudden surge of energy for physical activity.

Through awareness and understanding, mental fitness practices can help you better manage and reduce stress, especially the unhealthful kind that provides little, if any, health benefit.

These days, the stress that once helped you survive in the wild is now threatening your health and well-being, because many of the perceived threats we now face are informational and seemingly inescapable, that keep us in a constant state of stress.

This is all by human design. The stress induced by much of the media, entertainment, news, and apps we consume triggers your stress response for a reason. By keeping your amygdala in an activated state, your prefrontal cortex is inhibited that, in turn inhibits your critical thinking, impulse control, and emotional regulation, making it easier to unconsciously influence your thoughts, feelings, and behaviors emotionally.

It's a lot like telling someone who's swimming, "Be careful! There's a shark in the water!"

Does that calm the swimmer's stress response? Absolutely not.

Does it help the swimmer know exactly where the shark is to avoid it? Nope.

What it does do is triggers their stress response to panic and worry about the threat they cannot see, until they find it, or know for sure that they're safe from it.

When there's a threat we can't see, we can try to find it either face-to-face or from a safe place (i.e., media). If it's a serious enough threat, we might even go hunting for it ourselves, until we find it, to get rid of it.

Of course media developers and producers know this too.

The next time you see or hear a news headline that goes something like this, "There's something that might kill you... tune in at eleven to find out!" you'll know that it's a deliberate attempt to trigger your unconscious stress response to inhibit your critical thinking, impulse control, and emotional regulation, that leaves you in a stressed state until you find out what the threat is.

We even fight with people we love when our unconscious stress response is triggered, even when fighting causes more harm than good. It's hard to behave calmly and rationally when our unconscious stress response is triggered because it also inhibits the powers of our conscious mind, which is why practicing emotional awareness and stress management are so important.

In this technological age, the human nervous system is being continuously overwhelmed by endless amounts of threats and stress, to which the human brain has not yet evolved or adapted to maintain a healthful balanced state. The best your brain might do is adapt or acclimate to the chronic high level of stress, and even begin to anticipate it, at which point your stress threshold may increase as your nervous system becomes desensitized. This is often why we seek out stressful relationships when we've been raised in a stressful home environment, to balance our external environment with our internal environment.

If you haven't personally experienced burnout (yet), you likely know someone who has or is on the verge.

While more and more people are feeling fed up with the unhealthy and unsustainable stress levels of modern life, the truth is that burnout isn't just about feeling overwhelmed, but also under-cared for, under-respected, under-valued, and under-appreciated, with little hope, help, and healing—that triggers our unconscious stress response, flooding our system with cortisol and impairing our prefrontal cortex and parasympathetic nervous system.

With so much stress, strife, and struggle constantly happening around the world, we aren't just dealing with the compounded stresses of our immediate environment either. We are also processing global stresses that are societal in nature, far beyond our individual control, that add even more stress, tension, tragedy, grief, and trauma to our already maxed-out neurological system.

This applies to every human being who consumes stressful media and information on top of the stresses they face in their personal life.

The unhealthiest part is that with little to no control or solution, there is rarely anything we can do to fight or flee— other than fight with or flee from each other. We might fight or protest, choose to move or isolate ourselves, or tune-out. In other cases, we might even freeze, emotionally paralyzed by the overwhelming nature of the stress that we can neither fight nor flee.

However we physically respond to stresses we cannot control, we are highly susceptible to developing mental, emotional, and behavioral health conditions as a neurological response to toxic levels of stress that we cannot solve, fight, or flee. In a sense, it's like an energy surge in our brain that has no way to relieve itself, and ultimately harms our internal systems.

The best you can do is make your brain health a priority by managing stress within your neurological and physiological capabilities, that includes turning off stressful media and devices to optimize your well-being by feeling and doing your best—even when your best might change each day.

STRENGTH & ENDURANCE

Level Four: Strength & Endurance

☐ **Listen to music to relax or motivate your brain**

☐ **Reward healthful behaviors you need to repeat!**

☐ **Practice love and forgiveness**

☐ **Identify your "why"—what or who inspires you?**

Strength and endurance are the ultimate fitness levels to maintain, supported by the essential practices of balance, flexibility, and rest and recovery. There's a neurological reason why fitness practices do not start with strength and endurance, but rather build up to it.

Mental strength and endurance involve developing the skills you need to manage and navigate your unconscious stress response to optimize your thoughts, feelings, and behaviors, to achieve healthful outcomes.

We often associate strength and endurance with power, and by now you know that power is really about one's ability to influence. Therefore, true empowerment really comes from believing in yourself and your abilities, to influence your own health and well-being as well as being a healthful influence for others.

Strength is your ability to perform or do the work to achieve your goals, that requires a balanced, flexible, and resilient neurological foundation.

Endurance is your ability to continue the work to achieve your goals by maintaining your motivation over time, even as your goals might change, reset, or restart, as you keep taking one step forward to get where you want to go.

Part of building your strength and endurance is learning how to set (and reset) realistic and achievable goals, including realistic and achievable expectations for yourself and others.

Seeking support when you need it is as essential for developing mental strength as it is physical strength. Just as any seasoned bodybuilder seeks the support of a "spotter" when lifting a heavy weight to prevent injury and promote healthful development, seeking support is an important part of developing mental strength as well.

29 MUSIC, MEDIA, AND ENTERTAINMENT

Do you have a favorite song, movie, game, or TV show? What is it that you like about it?

More specifically, how does it make you feel?

What we like or find entertaining has to do with our unconscious emotional response and the related neurochemicals produced, that can be different for different people.

Marketers and advertisers sure know how to identify what drives people to act, consume, spend, and give—namely, what triggers our unconscious sense of reward and stress response.

Representation in media also matters, for all people. As much as we struggle with the ramifications of unconscious bias, it is also an essential part of our stress response system and survival instinct.

For better or worse, we feel safest (less stressed) with those who we perceive as familiar, someone with whom we can relate on some level. When we don't believe someone understands our feelings or experience, or we fear they will judge us or have a bias or prejudice against us, we can lose that essential sense of safety and trust that reduces our stress response and plays such a critical part in mental health, healing, and well-being—to feel and do our best.

For all of these reasons, mental fitness is often less about "what" you consume (that's often out of your control) and more about "how" you process what you consume through all of your senses—inside and out—and the healthful practices you can do to reduce stress, to feel and do your best.

When you are easy to trigger, you are also easy to influence and manipulate (which is why fitness might also be considered a form of self-defense or conflict management).

Your thoughts and feelings should not be dictated by the headlines of the day, curated by digital algorithms, commercial advertisers, corporations, or politicians intent on influencing and manipulating your thoughts, feelings, and behaviors, for the sake of their own power and profit.

While there can be a lot of unhealthy influences in the media you consume, there can also be a lot of healthful benefits to the media you consume as well. As with everything, the real skill to develop is the ability to differentiate healthful from unhealthful based on whether it influences your thoughts, feelings, and behaviors in healthful ways, to achieve healthful outcomes.

Music is another form of media that can affect your brain and body in a number of ways. The study of neurological and physiological effects of music on your brain and body is also a growing and fascinating area of research.

Music can trigger long-term memories and emotions, speed up or slow down your heart rate, help you express and process unconscious emotions, help you feel socially connected and understood, and even stimulate a greater sense of hope and motivation, by the way your brain and body absorb and process rhythmic and tonal sound waves, as well as lyrics through your neurological senses.

As with anything you consume, it's important to be aware of how music and other media influence your thoughts, feelings, and behaviors, to determine for yourself what you need to feel and do your best.

30 MORE REWARD, LESS PUNISHMENT

There's so much that influences your thoughts, feelings, worries, concerns, hopes, and dreams, that all influence your perceptions and behaviors, that impact your health and well-being, and the health and well-being of others.

Traumatic experiences make it hard to shake that unconscious fear of the unknown. When you realize that not knowing is what makes you the most vulnerable and puts you at greater risk, you quickly learn that contrary to the cultural cliché, ignorance is not bliss.

The brain becomes hyper aware of any potential threat, even when there's no explicit indication of a threat. Your unconscious stress response still makes you alert and suspicious. All your brain knows is that something hurtful happened when you let your guard down, so you keep your guard up. You might perceive everyone (or a specific type of person) as a potential threat to avoid. When others use your ignorance against you, you quickly learn that the element of surprise is the greatest weapon, and to remain vigilant.

Of course that's also the root of unconscious bias and

hypervigilance, that's not a healthful mental state to stay in, especially when you're struggling with other mental or emotional conditions like anxiety, grief, or depression.

Challenging one's unconscious stress response can also be perceived as a threat. Therefore, efforts to lower someone's stress response might actually have the opposite effect, and actually increased their perception of danger if they let down their guard. Thanks to how the human brain works, attempting to help someone who is in a defensive mental state can still be perceived as a threat to their personal safety and well-being, further triggering their unconscious stress response.

While it's so easy and obvious to accept help from someone we trust when the powers of our prefrontal cortex are fully functional, to comprehend and think critically, it can be extremely difficult to trust someone when our unconscious stress response takes over. When our unconscious biases and stress response kick in, we can easily perceive someone who is lending a helping hand as a threat. In that instant, our brain struggles to rationalize our emotions and defend ourselves.

This is also why confirmation bias is so hard to correct when we perceive someone as a threat.

When the person we perceive as a threat does not respond in a threatening way, we can perceive their non-threatening response as devious or deceitful, since that is the perception we already have of them. We may believe they are trying to manipulate us by seeming friendly and trustworthy, trying to get us to let down our guard to leave us vulnerable to their attack. It's this increase in own anger and aggression that reinforces our own unconscious bias, perception, and stress response.

This is also often what bothers a bully the most, when the one being bullied does not react or seem hurt by their abuse (even when we are). Your non-response might at first make the bully even angrier and more upset, since you are threatening their sense of power and influence over you, that makes them feel superior and better about themselves.

Do you remember the last time you were teased or bullied? Did you try to ignore them, to not let them see how much it bothered you? Do you remember how the person who was teasing or bullying you responded?

In many cases, when the person teasing or bullying doesn't get the defensive stress response they want, it can increase their unconscious stress response when your conscious effort to resist their attack is perceived as fighting back with mental strength. In response, they may at first try to tease and bully you even MORE (ugh).

However, if their attempts continue to fail, with your continued conscious effort to regulate your emotions and stress response (as badly as you might want to call them a hurtful name and fight back!), then their perception of you as an easy target is no longer being reinforced, and eventually changes. They may finally change their abusive behavior when they no longer get the dopamine rush they crave from your defensive stress response, and might actually try being your "friend"—likely in an attempt to develop a different kind of emotional influence over you again, so please beware that an unhealed person does not heal unless they do the work to heal themselves.

Healing unconscious biases really takes a lot of conscious effort, time, and patience (an emotional strength), through repeated nonthreatening experiences that gradually balance our stress response and perception by engaging the prefrontal cortex. Since our unconscious stress response is so strong, however, any improvement can be easily shattered by another threatening experience that reinforces our unconscious bias again.

There is an enormous amount of invisible stress, fear, pain, and worry that most of us carry inside at all times, not to mention the various mental health and neurological conditions that so many of us are dealing with invisibly as well, that makes dealing with stress and pain that much harder.

You can apply this neurological phenomenon directly to how our society has historically dealt with crime and punishment as well, and why our system is struggling. When "corrective action" focuses on punishing behaviors, it simply triggers the unconscious stress response to avoid punishment (i.e., not getting caught).

When we focus solely on punishment alone in the name of crime prevention, there is actually no proactive preventive quality about it. We don't actually motivate, reward, or reinforce the repetition of healthful and lawful behaviors since those are driven by the prefrontal cortex that becomes inhibited by imbalance, trauma, or an otherwise overactive amygdala.

Punishment simply reinforces the stress response that motivates us to avoid punishment, whether that means fighting, fleeing, or freezing when caught. We might comply at first, in order to avoid punishment, but we are not actually developing more healthful behaviors—just avoidance. This is very much the same way any other animal that is afraid of its handler may learn to comply with their demands in order to prevent punishment, and why that animal is more likely to attack their handler when they turn their back.

Our fear of pain and punishment might be strong enough to make us not want to do something—when the costs don't outweigh the benefits.

This doesn't just apply to criminal punishment either.

We are also often punished just for being our authentic selves, when how we think or behave does not comply with those in positions of power, influence, and authority. The idea of personal empowerment might actually be perceived as a threat by groups or individuals in positions of power, due to their own unconscious stress response.

When the perception remains that someone is our enemy, no amount of telling them they are wrong will change that.

This is also why continual threats and intimidation during interrogations can lead to false confessions, in order to get out of that threatening and stressful state that inhibits our critical thinking, comprehension, and problem-solving abilities—when all we want to do is flee and get out of there.

What's needed is a sense of trust, to lower their stress response, to engage their prefrontal cortex, to promote healthful neurological and physiological activity that allows them to process information in a non-threatening way, that allows their perception to naturally change and alleviate cognitive dissonance, by rebalancing their mental system.

31 LOVE AND FORGIVENESS

What does "love" mean to you? And what's the difference between "like" and "love"?

There are probably as many definitions for the word "love" as there are people on the planet, but for purposes of mental fitness, health and well-being, we'll define "love" as the desire for one to thrive and flourish—whether that's loving yourself or another person, place, thing, or animal.

With this definition in mind, the major difference between "like" and "love" would be in whether it helps one thrive, heal, and grow, or if the sentiment is purely for your own pleasure and enjoyment.

We tend to like things that bring us pleasure and enjoyment, but love is an emotional investment that comes with some emotional risk as well. When you want what's best for that which you love, you may need to lose it, let it go, or set it free, that may result in painful emotions related to grief.

For example, you might like hiking outside because it brings you pleasure, but you might harm nature in doing so, by disrupting or polluting the natural habitats of other animals. If you love nature, you might take extra precautions to not disrupt or pollute the natural environment. In order to protect nature, the area you love might even be closed off to hikers. This loss of an activity that brought you so much joy might make you sad, but also happy that it's being cared for and protected, so it can thrive and flourish long after you're able to enjoy it.

Why is it important to differentiate love from like in your mental fitness?

Your brain responds differently between the emotions of like and love, with a stronger neurochemical response related to love (namely oxytocin).

Love can feel deeply joyful as well as deeply painful. Love can be deeply healing when we focus more on what is best for the person, place, thing, or animal we love—including love for ourselves. Though it may feel painful to go through a divorce, or when a child leaves home, focusing on what's best for them to grow, thrive, and flourish can help reduce stress and engage your prefrontal cortex, that is part of the healing process that allows you to grow, thrive, and flourish as well.

Of course these healthful outcomes are only achieved when we have the mental fitness skills to understand and regulate our emotions and unconscious stress response.

When pleasure turns into displeasure, disgust, disappointment, fear or pain, our feelings can quickly turn into intense dislike, or even hate, depending on the intensity of neurochemical activity from our unconscious stress response.

This is when the practice of "unconditional" love and forgiveness are most important, to maintain our desire for one to thrive and flourish even when our unconscious stress response is triggered.

Even when love involves the fear and pain of loss or letting go, we can achieve the most healthful outcomes when we focus on what's needed to thrive and flourish.

Our sense of competition and desire to be "the winner" (or at least better than the one that hurt us) can make the practice of unconditional love and forgiveness even harder by compounding our stress level.

Similar to those intense feelings of love, when we proclaim someone as "the best" or superior to others in some way, it's only a relative judgment based on our own perception. We are only comparing what we know, not what we don't. Who knows if there is someone else in a remote part of the world who is even better, who may never have the opportunity to try, learn, or be discovered?

Many of us were taught that to become successful means you need to be "the best," which instills a sense of competition and also antagonism—that sense of "us vs. them."

In reality, often the most successful people are not "the best" by themselves, but are those who have the ability and influence to find others to help them—to leverage diverse abilities that are stronger together, to succeed collectively.

This is also why "divide and conquer" is a strategy, based on the fact that we are stronger when we work together and support each other, and the easiest way to conquer people is to divide them.

Unfortunately, our competitive culture that rewards individual success and individual contribution teaches us the opposite— that we are stronger when we are apart and competing with each other.

At the end of the day, achievement is not a matter of knowing it all yourself, but the ability to connect with others who know different pieces to help put all of the pieces together.

Likewise, success is not a matter of winners and losers, but teaching and learning through successes and failures, to grow as we go.

This is also the power in forgiveness, that is not about condoning or forgetting what caused you pain, but allowing yourself to feel and do your best by healing your mind neurologically. By reducing stress and tension, resentment and hostility, you can reduce the rumination that continually triggers your amygdala and floods your system with unhealthy levels of cortisol.

Contrary to the popular phrase "forgive and forget," forgetting has nothing to do with forgiveness. You cannot wipe memories from your neurology simply by wanting it. This notion of being able to control your memories further contributes to the shame and stigma that get in the way of proper mental healthcare. It is neither healthful nor realistic to expect someone who has been emotionally traumatized to just wipe their traumatic memories and experiences away, when they are burned deep in their neurology that also impacts their physiology.

There is an evolutionary reason to remembering the things that hurt you—so you don't repeat them and get hurt again. Learning from our pains and mistakes is an important and healthful part of life. There is also a reason why, by consciously practicing the emotional state of forgiveness, memories might fade over time when you don't ruminate and neurologically reinforce them over and over again.

This is in part why we say "time heals all wounds." Over time, with less and less repetition and reinforcement, you may not remember the experience as clearly that at one time caused you so much pain. You might get to a point when you can remember how hurtful the experience was, to share your painful experience with others, without triggering such a severe unconscious stress response.

When we hold onto pain and anger, it impairs our health and well-being in many ways. We might even derive some sense of power and pleasure from the cortisol and adrenaline as part of the stress response that helps numb the pain. We might use our stress response as a source of motivation as well. Chronic stress can contribute to a number of health risk factors, including high blood pressure, heart disease, obesity, anxiety, depression, drug abuse, and increased risk of suicide.

The mental and emotional practice of forgiveness is one way to reduce the toxic effects of pain, anger, and stress by lowering the level of cortisol in your system, to rebalance your metabolic and nervous systems, allowing your brain and body to heal, and improve your health and well-being. The healing process is always relative to the amount of pain you are carrying, your neurological state, and the amount of healing you have to do, that may require more specialized care and support from a licensed therapist.

32 MAINTAINING MOTIVATION

"JUST DO IT" might be a classic ad slogan, but why do we need to be told do something that is healthy and beneficial for us?

It's not a matter of "willpower." That old "bootstraps" theory of motivation basically implies you should be able to do it all on your own, whether you have the essential healthful influences you need or not.

While it might seem much easier (and less stressful) to believe we have control of every thought, feeling, and behavior as a result of "willpower," the theory of willpower also contributes to much of the shame, blame, and stigma that surrounds brain health and mental well-being, and prevents people from seeking and receiving the mental health services and support they need.

When you've lost hope and don't believe you can do it (whatever "it" is), you need more than just being told to "just do it" on your own. Maybe you've been told by others that you can't, or you've already tried and failed, or you have a mental health condition due to a trauma, illness, impairment, or imbalance that drains your energy.

It's neither healthful nor realistic to tell someone to just get over their grief, anxiety, addiction, eating disorder, or depression either.

When we say "just do it," we're basically ignoring brain health, development, and function, contributing to the stigma that surrounds mental healthcare as well. This is but one example of the culture we've created that stigmatizes mental health challenges and conditions by believing we should have control over it, if you just wish it and want it enough.

Of course this is not the reality of the human brain.

To feel motivated, you first need a sense of hope that is influenced neurologically by everything in and around you.

At the very core of nearly every goal is a basic belief or hope of how achieving that goal will make you feel—whether that's feeling seen, respected, valued, accomplished, safe, loved, desired, or some other benefit or good feeling, that makes it seem worthwhile.

When you're told to "fake it 'til you make it," it basically reinforces your self-perception that you can't, that's neither healthful nor authentic. There are many ways to improve your self-perception without resorting to lying or faking it.

The first step to achieving anything is really the perception that it is possible, that allows you to believe you can. Your perception is influenced by all that's in and around you— including your thoughts, feelings, information, relationships, environment, nutrition, and body chemistry.

Rather than lying to yourself and others, it's more healthful (and sustainable) to develop your self-perception by finding healthful influences, including those who believe in your abilities. It's not a sign of weakness to acknowledge your fears and insecurities, to face them head-on. It's actually a sign of strength, when you can overcome those fears that get in your way of feeling and doing your best, by navigating your unconscious stress response in a more healthful way (realizing that lying also makes your stress response worse).

While emotional regulation and impulse control are powers that a fully developed and healthy brain can generally do, the prefrontal cortex that powers them can still be inhibited when our unconscious stress response is triggered by fear, worry, panic, or otherwise impaired by a neurological disorder or mental health condition.

It is true that maintaining behaviors are much easier once you get started, after taking that first important step, so there is obvious healthful intent. Your unconscious stress response can be a very effective "motivator" in the short-term, by releasing cortisol and adrenaline that prepare your body for "fight or flight," but can also put you at greater risk of unhealthy outcomes.

When someone tells you (or you tell yourself) to "JUST DO IT," you might feel that burst of motivation (i.e., cortisol and adrenaline) that motivates you in that moment. When you rely on your stress response as a source of motivation, however, it likely won't work as well after the third or fourth time, as your brain adapts to the unconscious neurochemical effect, and it starts to wear off. You might then need to increase the stress level (maybe by someone shouting at you or calling you names, or procrastinating more and more) in order to achieve the same neurochemical stress response.

Since your stress response is triggered by your amygdala, your prefrontal cortex also becomes inhibited. Relying on your stress response may make you more neurologically dependent on someone else telling you what to think or do, thereby increasing their power and reducing yours. As your unconscious stress response fuels your motivation, you also feel rewarded when the stress subsides—reinforcing your aversion to stress. This is why fitness programs that rely on stress as a motivator can be difficult to maintain—while your motivated by the stress, you also want to avoid it.

The neurochemical fluctuation that requires heightened levels of cortisol and adrenaline also puts wear and tear on your cells and organs, altering your metabolism by inhibiting the "rest, digest, and repair" state of your parasympathetic nervous system. So if weight management is one of your fitness goals, being motivated by stress is often counterproductive. You might experience irregular weight fluctuations, an upset stomach, heart palpitations, acne, skin rash, or any number of other long-term physical and mental health conditions associated with chronic stress (e.g., heart disease, anxiety, depression, etc.).

You know that feeling when you care about something so much that it turns into worry and panic? That is when your prefrontal cortex triggers your amygdala.

As you work toward a goal, and time seems to fly, your sense of passion and purpose can quickly turn into worry when you don't allow time to rest, rebalance, and refocus—when you put extra stress and pressure on yourself believing it will motivate you and do some good (the trickery of our unconscious stress response!).

It's no joke that maintaining your focus, critical thinking, and creativity (powered by your prefrontal cortex) can be a tremendous challenge without managing the stress that comes from your immense sense of caring, passion, and purpose, that can quickly trigger worry and panic in your amygdala when you don't make your mental fitness a priority.

It's important to practice getting enough quality sleep, drinking plenty of water, eating nutrient-rich foods, taking time to move and stretch your body, listening to uplifting music, being in the moment to celebrate each step (even when your destination seems miles away), setting healthful boundaries (that includes the ability to say "NO" to unhealthful demands and expectations), and limiting stressful media and news that you can do nothing about—to increase energy in your prefrontal cortex, to focus on the things you can.

Since blame and shame require less neurological energy and effort as an unconscious stress response (powered by the amygdala), it's much easier neurologically for the brain to blame and judge people for not having the "willpower" to behave in healthful or socially acceptable ways, rather than making a conscious effort to empathize and understand what drive behaviors neurologically and physiologically in the brain.

It's not a lack of "willpower" that holds us back, but a lack of hope, and lack of awareness of how our brains and bodies work. The smallest sense of hope can change our trajectory by reducing your unconscious stress response to engage our prefrontal cortex, fueling the smallest sense of motivation to wake up, to take one step, to take on the day, to find the healthful influences and support we need.

Maintaining motivation is really a skill that requires continual practice, support, and adjustment, that starts with a very simple, yet often difficult, practice of engaging your prefrontal cortex to comprehend and understand by asking yourself, "Why?" as well as "Why not?"

Even when you feel tired and hopeless, you can give yourself a little neurochemical boost by understanding why something is important and worthwhile to try, to give you the smallest trickle of energy you need to take the next important step, no matter how big or small.

Asking "Why?" as a way to engage and understand (rather than deny or deflect) is one healthful way to maintain your motivation by engaging your prefrontal cortex, to calm your amygdala, to reduce cortisol and rebalance your system, by being consciously aware of the purpose and reward of what it is you want to do or achieve.

Like every other part of your biology, the neurology and physiology in your brain are in constant flux—constantly absorbing, processing, adapting, healing, and detoxifying from all you consume and experience. Just as your brain and body need to rebalance, so must your sense of motivation.

If you are struggling to ask and understand, then that may be a neurological sign of a more serious mental health condition that requires more specialized care and support than you can provide yourself on your own, to help recover or rebalance your system to a more healthful state.

This is absolutely nothing to feel ashamed about, only to understand about yourself as a neurochemical being. Asking, "Why is this hard for me?" is as important and valid to ask about your mental abilities as much as your physical abilities, to optimize both your physical and mental health and well-being.

Even when you don't have all of the answers, the real aim is to engage your brain in a healthful way to stay motivated and curious, not hopeless and afraid. There is real power in wonder and exploration, in asking questions and seeking answers, in caring for your brain and body to optimize your mental and physical abilities, to find solutions and achieve what you want to achieve, to get the most out the life you have. When an answer is not available or easy to find, that's when it can help to rely on faith to have hope, that is also an opportunity to keep asking, thinking, creating, exploring, and discovering—

not a reason to stop.

Your sense of hope can be easily dashed by the unconscious forces of stress—from shame, intimidation, misinformation, or other unhealthy influences that impact your perception of what's possible and worthwhile by triggering your unconscious stress response.

We all need a bit of encouragement and positive affirmation to fuel our motivation—to get those healthful neurochemicals flowing that energize and motivate us with a sense of hope and optimism. While feeling hopeful is a powerful force, it's also a very fragile state that requires conscious effort and support to maintain, to prevent your unconscious stress response from triggering unhealthful thoughts, feelings, and behaviors.

So instead of being hard on yourself for lacking motivation (that triggers an unconscious stress response), focus on finding, creating, and maintaining those healthful influences that inspire and motivate you—that might change as you go too.

Here are a few healthful influences that could help you maintain your motivation in healthful ways:

- A mentor or role model who can help shape your perception of what's possible
- A warm hug or chat with a friend that helps reduce stress
- A nutritious breakfast that nourishes your brain and body
- Enough quality sleep to rest and rebalance your neurological and physiological system
- A physical workout or walk outside
- A game or creative project
- Volunteering or community service
- Words of wisdom or encouragement

Mental fitness is really about building wisdom, by applying what you learn to your own life in a healthful way, to help you navigate all of the wonderful, painful, challenging, rewarding, and often confusing experiences in life—including love and loss, and facing your fears.

The exciting part is that there is still so much to be learned and discovered, that you must experience and learn for yourself, by living your life, as you navigate the challenges you face every day.

Be sure to use your power of influence, by sharing your sense of hope and motivation to influence those around you, to help foster and fuel a community of healthful influencers who help maintain motivation and healthful habits to achieve healthful outcomes for all!

MY BRAIN CAN'T POOP

THIS IS THE BEGINNING

I hope this beginner's guide to mental fitness for humans helps make better sense of yourself and others, to shed some light on why life can feel so wonderful and challenging too. Living life without understanding the inner workings of yourself and others can make it even harder, which is why focusing on mental fitness is so important to navigating life in a healthful way.

Understanding and awareness are what help us navigate. Life can sometimes feel like we're being pushed in the deep end without first learning how to swim. So in a way, you can consider this book a swimming lesson. Much like swimming in uncharted water, the trick to thriving in life is to not panic, so you can focus on what you need to do to stay afloat until you reach land or help arrives.

Of course these skills are easier said than done when we aren't provided the time or opportunity to practice and develop them. If there is one skill I wish we taught in schools, it is how to navigate the ups and downs of life that constantly change as we age and grow—as our brains age and change too.

When you know enough to maintain hope and stay afloat, you are better able to maintain your drive and motivation to get where you need to go, with the knowledge of what you can do to get there.

I hope you continue to learn and remain curious as you develop the knowledge, skills, and abilities you need to feel and do your best, that begins by taking care of your brain.

MY BRAIN CAN'T POOP

ABOUT THE AUTHOR

Scott Mikesh is an award-winning business leader and mental fitness instructor with more than twenty years of experience in applied psychology, health and wellness, communications and design, program management, and diversity, equity, and inclusion. Scott is the Founder and Instructor of 4D Fit Mental Fitness based in St. Paul, Minnesota, where he currently resides with his husband Nick, a dog named Nela, a fish named Flounder, and a tarantula named Barb. To learn more about Scott and 4D Fit, please visit www.4dfit.net.

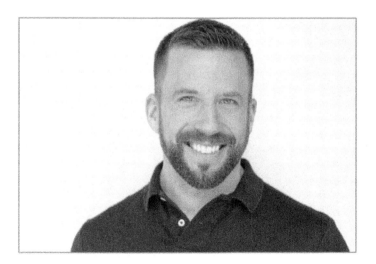

Made in the USA
Monee, IL
08 February 2022